EFFORTLESS CARNIVORE DIET FOR BEGINNERS

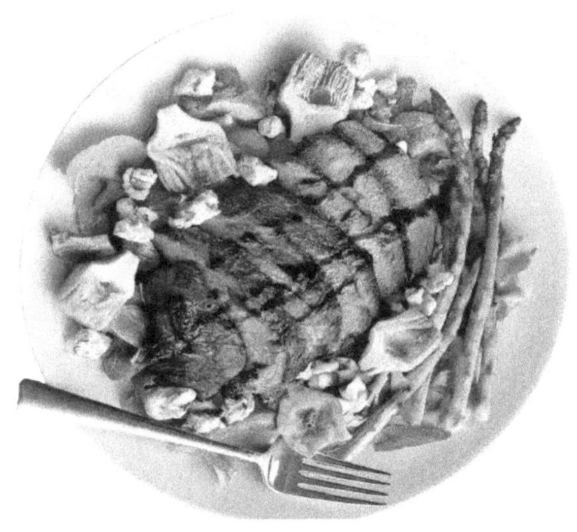

Delicious Recipes for a Healthy Transformation

Leroy Johnson

Table of Contents

INTRODUCTION

Welcome, fellow meat enthusiasts, to a beginner's guide to the carnivore diet. If you've found yourself here, you're likely intrigued by the prospect of harnessing the power of meat for optimal health and vitality. Well, you're in the right place. In this comprehensive cookbook, we'll embark on a journey to explore the ins and outs of the carnivore lifestyle, from its humble beginnings to its modern resurgence as a powerhouse dietary approach.

Unraveling the Mysteries of the Carnivore Diet

Let's address the elephant in the room—what exactly is the carnivore diet, and why has it captured the attention of so many health-conscious individuals? At its core, the carnivore diet is a dietary regimen that emphasizes the consumption of animal products while eschewing plant-based foods. While this may seem perplexing to some, proponents of the carnivore lifestyle argue that it offers a myriad of benefits, ranging from weight loss and increased energy to improved mental clarity and digestive health.

Dispelling Myths and Misconceptions

Before we delve into the delicious recipes and practical tips that await you in these pages, it's crucial to address some common misconceptions surrounding the carnivore diet. Contrary to popular belief, a carnivore diet is not synonymous with reckless meat consumption or nutritional imbalance. When approached mindfully and responsibly, the carnivore lifestyle can provide all the essential nutrients your body needs to thrive.

The Science behind the Carnivore Lifestyle

You may be wondering: what scientific evidence supports the efficacy of the carnivore diet? While the carnivore lifestyle may seem counterintuitive in a world inundated with messages promoting plant-based diets, numerous studies and anecdotal reports have highlighted its potential benefits. From improved metabolic health to reduced inflammation, the carnivore diet has garnered attention for its ability to positively impact various aspects of well-being.

Take a step on Your Carnivore Journey

Now that we've laid the groundwork, it's time for you to embark on your carnivore journey. Whether you're a seasoned meat lover or a curious newcomer, this cookbook is designed to meet you where you are and guide you every step of the way. From stocking your kitchen with carnivore-friendly ingredients to mastering mouthwatering recipes, consider this your roadmap to success in the world of meat-centric eating.

The Ultimate Resource for Carnivores

As you flip through the pages of this cookbook, you'll discover a treasure trove of culinary inspiration and practical advice. Each recipe has been meticulously crafted to showcase the versatility and deliciousness of meat, proving that the carnivore lifestyle is anything but restrictive. So, grab your apron, sharpen your knives, and prepare to savor the incredible flavors that await you on your carnivore journey.

The ultimate carnivore diet is not just a dietary approach—it's a lifestyle. By embracing the simplicity and satiety of meat-centric eating, you're not only nourishing your body but also reconnecting with the primal essence of human nutrition. So, dive in, explore, and revel in the abundance of flavors that await you in these pages. Your carnivore adventure starts now.

CHAPTER 1: Understanding the Carnivore diet

What is a Carnivore diet?

The carnivore diet, often hailed as a radical departure from conventional dietary wisdom, is a nutritional approach centered on the consumption of animal products while excluding plant-based foods. At its core, the carnivore diet is a return to our ancestral roots—a primal embrace of the foods that sustained our earliest human ancestors.

Unlike other dietary regimens that emphasize a balance of macronutrients from various food groups, the carnivore diet places a singular focus on animal-derived foods. This includes meat, fish, poultry, eggs, and certain dairy products, with an emphasis on high-quality, nutrient-dense sources. By eliminating plant-based foods such as fruits, vegetables, grains, and legumes, proponents of the carnivore diet argue that it simplifies the digestive process, reduces inflammation, and promotes optimal health and well-being.

Contrary to popular belief, the carnivore diet is not a license to indulge in an endless feast of steak and bacon. Instead, it encourages mindful consumption of a diverse array of animal products, including organ meats, bone broth, and fatty cuts of meat. By prioritizing nutrient density and bioavailability, the carnivore diet aims to provide all the essential nutrients our bodies need for optimal function, without the need for supplementation or fortified foods.

While the carnivore diet may seem perplexing or even controversial to some, it has gained traction in recent years due to a growing body of anecdotal evidence and scientific research supporting its potential benefits. From improved metabolic health and weight management to enhanced mental clarity and athletic performance, individuals who embrace the carnivore lifestyle often report a myriad of positive outcomes.

In essence, the carnivore diet represents a departure from conventional dietary norms—a return to a simpler, more primal way of eating that celebrates the nutrient-rich bounty of the animal kingdom. Whether you're a seasoned carnivore or a curious newcomer, exploring the carnivore diet offers an opportunity to reconnect with our evolutionary heritage and rediscover the transformative power of meat-centric eating.

What to eat during a Carnivore Diet

Embarking on a carnivore diet means embracing a culinary adventure centered solely on animal-derived foods. While the simplicity of this approach may initially seem perplexing, rest assured that the carnivore diet offers a surprisingly diverse array of delicious options to tantalize your taste buds and nourish your body.

1. **High-Quality Meats**: At the heart of the carnivore diet lies a plethora of meats, each offering its own unique flavor profile and nutritional benefits. Indulge in juicy steaks, tender roasts, succulent ribs, and flavorful burgers made from beef, lamb, pork, and venison. Opt for grass-fed, pasture-raised, or wild-caught options whenever possible to maximize nutrient density and minimize exposure to antibiotics and hormones.

2. **Poultry and Game**: Expand your palate with a variety of poultry and game meats, including chicken, turkey, duck, quail, pheasant, and game birds. Whether roasted, grilled, or smoked, these lean sources of protein provide a delicious alternative to traditional red meats while offering essential nutrients like B vitamins and iron.

3. **Fish and Seafood**: Dive into the ocean's bounty with an assortment of fish and seafood options. From fatty fish like salmon, mackerel, and sardines to shellfish such as shrimp, crab, and lobster, there's no

shortage of marine delicacies to enjoy on a carnivore diet. Rich in omega-3 fatty acids, protein, and minerals, fish and seafood offer a nutrient-packed addition to your carnivore repertoire.

4. **Eggs**: Versatile and nutrient-dense, eggs are a carnivore staple that can be enjoyed in countless ways. Whether scrambled, fried, poached, or hard-boiled, eggs provide a convenient source of protein, vitamins, and minerals. Opt for pasture-raised or omega-3 enriched eggs for added nutritional benefits.

5. **Dairy Products (Optional)**: While some carnivores choose to exclude dairy from their diets, others may incorporate dairy products such as cheese, butter, and heavy cream in moderation. Look for high-quality, full-fat dairy options from grass-fed animals to ensure optimal nutrient content and minimize potential allergens.

6. **Organ Meats**: Don't overlook the nutritional powerhouse that is organ meats. Liver, heart, kidney, and other organ meats are packed with essential nutrients like vitamins A, D, E, and K, as well as B vitamins, iron, and zinc. Incorporate organ meats into your carnivore diet to reap their myriad health benefits and add depth of flavor to your meals.

By focusing on these nutrient-dense animal-derived foods, you can craft a satisfying and nourishing carnivore diet that promotes optimal health and vitality. Experiment with different cuts, cooking methods, and flavor combinations to keep your carnivore journey exciting and bursting with flavor. Remember to prioritize high-quality, ethically sourced ingredients whenever possible to ensure the best possible outcomes for both your health and the planet.

What not to eat during Carnivore Diet

While the carnivore diet may seem straightforward in its emphasis on animal-derived foods, it's equally important to understand what to avoid to ensure optimal results and adherence to the dietary principles. Here, we'll explore the foods that are typically excluded from a carnivore diet, along with the rationale behind these exclusions.

1. **Plant-Based Foods**: In the realm of carnivore cuisine, there exists a striking omission—plant-based foods. This encompasses a wide array of culinary delights, such as fruits, vegetables, grains, legumes, nuts, seeds, and plant oils. The rationale behind this exclusion lies in the desire to simplify the digestive process and eliminate potential sources of anti-nutrients, allergens, and digestive irritants found in many plant foods. While fruits and vegetables are commonly touted as essential components of a healthy diet, proponents of the carnivore lifestyle

argue that the nutrients found in these foods can be adequately obtained from animal-derived sources.

2. **Processed Foods**: Another category of foods to avoid on a carnivore diet is processed foods, including but not limited to refined grains, sugars, artificial sweeteners, preservatives, and additives. These highly processed foods are often devoid of nutritional value and may contribute to inflammation, metabolic dysfunction, and other health issues. By prioritizing whole, unprocessed animal-derived foods, carnivores can optimize their nutrient intake and support overall health and well-being.

3. **Plant-Based Substitutes**: In recent years, the market for plant-based substitutes has exploded, offering alternatives to traditional animal-derived foods such as meat, dairy, and eggs. While these products may appeal to individuals following vegetarian or vegan diets, they have no place in a carnivore diet. Plant-based substitutes are typically

highly processed and may contain a variety of additives, fillers, and flavor enhancers that are incompatible with the principles of a carnivore diet.

4. **Grains and Legumes**: Grains and legumes, including wheat, rice, corn, oats, beans, lentils, and soy, are commonly avoided on a carnivore diet due to their high carbohydrate content and potential for digestive irritation. Additionally, grains and legumes contain anti-nutrients such as lectins, phytates, and gluten, which can impair nutrient absorption and contribute to gastrointestinal distress. By eliminating grains and legumes from their diets, carnivores can minimize digestive issues and optimize nutrient absorption.

5. **Sugary and Starchy Foods**: Sugary and starchy foods, including candy, pastries, bread, pasta, potatoes, and other high-carbohydrate foods, are off-limits on a carnivore diet. These foods can cause rapid spikes in blood sugar levels, leading to insulin resistance, inflammation, and metabolic dysfunction

over time. By focusing on animal-derived foods that are naturally low in carbohydrates and sugar, carnivores can maintain stable blood sugar levels and support metabolic health.

6. **Industrial Vegetable Oils**: Industrial vegetable oils, such as soybean oil, corn oil, canola oil, and sunflower oil, are commonly used in processed foods and cooking. However, these oils are high in omega-6 fatty acids and may promote inflammation and oxidative stress when consumed in excess. Instead, carnivores opt for natural sources of fat such as animal fats, butter, ghee, and tallow, which provide a healthier balance of omega-3 and omega-6 fatty acids.

By avoiding these foods and focusing on nutrient-dense animal-derived foods, carnivores can optimize their health and well-being while enjoying a delicious and satisfying diet. Remember, the key to success on a carnivore diet lies in simplicity, quality, and mindful eating.

Benefits of Carnivore Diet for Beginners

The carnivore diet, with its emphasis on animal-derived foods and the exclusion of plant-based foods, has garnered attention for its potential to promote optimal health and well-being. While this dietary approach may seem unconventional at first glance, proponents of the carnivore lifestyle tout a myriad of benefits that can be experienced by those who adopt it. Let's explore some of the key benefits of the carnivore diet and the science behind its efficacy.

1. ***Simplified Digestion***: One of the primary benefits of the carnivore diet is its ability to simplify the digestive process. By eliminating complex carbohydrates, fiber, and plant-based anti-nutrients, carnivores give their digestive systems a break and may experience reduced bloating, gas, and digestive discomfort. This simplified digestion allows the body to allocate more energy towards other physiological processes, such as tissue repair and metabolic function.

2. **_Improved Nutrient Absorption_**: Animal-derived foods are rich sources of essential nutrients such as protein, vitamins, minerals, and healthy fats. By focusing on nutrient-dense animal products, carnivores can optimize their nutrient intake and support overall health and vitality. Additionally, the absence of anti-nutrients found in many plant foods may enhance nutrient absorption and utilization, leading to improved nutrient status over time.

3. **_Enhanced Metabolic Health_**: The carnivore diet has been associated with improvements in various markers of metabolic health, including insulin sensitivity, blood sugar control, and lipid profiles. By minimizing carbohydrate intake and stabilizing blood sugar levels, carnivores may reduce their risk of insulin resistance, type 2 diabetes, and metabolic syndrome. Additionally, the high protein content of animal-derived foods can support muscle maintenance and metabolic rate, contributing to

improved body composition and weight management.

4. ***Reduced Inflammation***: Chronic inflammation is a common underlying factor in many chronic diseases, including heart disease, cancer, and autoimmune conditions. The carnivore diet's exclusion of potential inflammatory triggers found in plant-based foods may help reduce systemic inflammation and promote overall health. Additionally, the nutrient-rich nature of animal-derived foods provides essential building blocks for the body's anti-inflammatory pathways, further supporting a balanced inflammatory response.

5. ***Mental Clarity and Cognitive Function***: Many carnivores report improvements in mental clarity, focus, and cognitive function when following a meat-centric diet. The stable energy levels provided by animal-derived foods, combined with the absence of potential brain fog-inducing carbohydrates and anti-nutrients, may contribute to enhanced mental

performance and productivity. Additionally, the omega-3 fatty acids found in fatty fish and seafood have been shown to support brain health and cognitive function.

6. ***Increased Satiety and Weight Management:*** Animal-derived foods are naturally high in protein and healthy fats, both of which are highly satiating and can help curb cravings and promote feelings of fullness. By prioritizing protein and fat-rich foods, carnivores may naturally reduce their caloric intake and improve their body's ability to regulate hunger and appetite. This can lead to sustainable weight loss or maintenance over time, without the need for restrictive calorie counting or portion control.

The carnivore diet offers a compelling array of potential benefits for those who choose to embrace it. From simplified digestion and improved nutrient absorption to enhanced metabolic health and mental clarity, the carnivore lifestyle has the potential to transform both body and mind. While individual experiences may vary, many carnivores report experiencing profound improvements in their health and well-being when following this meat-centric approach to eating. As with any dietary regimen, it's essential to listen to your body, prioritize quality and variety, and consult with a healthcare professional before making any significant dietary changes.

Twenty (20) Shopping Ingredients list

1. **Grass-fed Beef**: Look for cuts like ribeye, sirloin, or ground beef to serve as the foundation of your carnivore meals. Grass-fed beef tends to be higher in omega-3 fatty acids and other nutrients compared to conventionally raised beef.

2. **Pasture-Raised Chicken**: Opt for pasture-raised chicken thighs, breasts, or whole chickens for a versatile protein option that can be roasted, grilled, or baked to perfection.

3. **Wild-Caught Fish**: Choose fatty fish like salmon, mackerel, or sardines, which are rich in omega-3 fatty acids and provide a flavorful addition to your carnivore diet.

4. **Pasture-Raised Pork**: Explore cuts like pork chops, tenderloin, or bacon from pasture-raised pigs for a delicious and nutrient-dense protein source.

5. **Organ Meats**: Incorporate nutrient-rich organ meats such as liver, heart, and kidney into your diet to boost your intake of essential vitamins and minerals.

6. **Eggs:** Stock up on pasture-raised eggs, which are a convenient and affordable source of high-quality protein and essential nutrients.

7. **Bone Broth**: Consider adding bone broth to your shopping list for its collagen, gelatin, and mineral content, which can support gut health and overall well-being.

8. **Butter or Ghee:** Choose grass-fed butter or ghee as a flavorful cooking fat to enhance the taste of your carnivore meals while providing beneficial fatty acids.

9. **Tallow or Lard**: Include animal fats like tallow or lard in your shopping cart for cooking and frying purposes, adding richness and flavor to your dishes.

10. **Cheese (optional):** If you tolerate dairy well, select high-quality, full-fat cheeses like cheddar, Gouda, or parmesan to enjoy in moderation as a carnivore-friendly snack or topping.

11. **Heavy Cream (optional)**: For those who include dairy in their carnivore diet, heavy cream can be used to add richness and creaminess to sauces, coffee, or desserts.

12. **Salt:** Choose a high-quality sea salt or pink Himalayan salt to season your carnivore meals and replenish electrolytes lost through sweating.

13. **Pepper (optional):** If you enjoy a bit of spice, consider adding black pepper to your shopping list for seasoning meats and adding depth of flavor.

14. **Mineral Water**: Stay hydrated with mineral water rich in electrolytes like magnesium, calcium, and potassium, which can support hydration and mineral balance.

15. **Liverwurst or Pate:** Incorporate liverwurst or pate into your diet as a convenient and nutrient-dense way to enjoy organ meats.

16. **Bacon**: Indulge in the savory goodness of bacon, which adds flavor and texture to any carnivore meal while providing a satisfying dose of protein and fat.

17. **Salami or Pepperoni**: Keep a selection of cured meats like salami or pepperoni on hand for quick and portable carnivore-friendly snacks.

18. **Beef Jerky**: Choose grass-fed beef jerky as a convenient and shelf-stable option for satisfying your carnivorous cravings on the go.

19. **Egg Yolks**: Don't discard those egg yolks! Include them in your carnivore meals for their rich flavor and nutrient content, including vitamins A, D, E, and K.

20. **Sardines in Olive Oil**: Add canned sardines in olive oil to your shopping list for a convenient and nutrient-rich snack or meal option packed with omega-3 fatty acids and protein.

CHAPTER 2: Carnivore Diet Breakfast

1. Carnivore Breakfast Sandwich

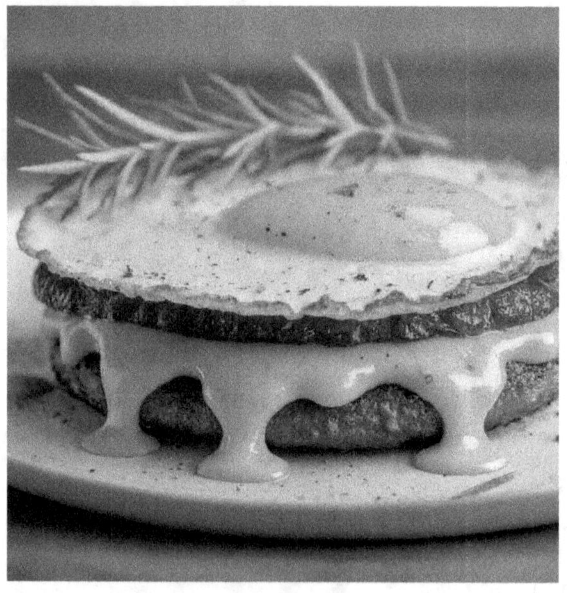

Preparation Time: 10 minutes

Cooking Time: 15 minutes

Ingredients:

- 2 beef patties

- 2 eggs, pasture-raised

- 2 slices cheddar cheese

- 4 slices bacon

- 1 tbsp. butter, tallow, or bacon grease

Instructions:

1. Cook the beef patties in a skillet over medium-high heat until cooked through, about 5-7 minutes per side.

2. In the same skillet, cook the bacon until crispy, about 3-5 minutes per side.

3. In a separate skillet, fry the eggs to your desired doneness.

4. Assemble the sandwich by placing one beef patty on the bottom, followed by a slice of cheese, an egg, and 2 slices of bacon. Top with the other beef patty and cheese slice.

5. Melt the butter, tallow, or bacon grease in the skillet and toast the sandwich until the cheese is melted and the bread is golden brown, about 2-3 minutes per side.

Nutritional Value (per serving):

- Calories: 448

- Fat: 36g

- Protein: 33g

- Carbohydrates: 0g

2. Carnivore Fat Bomb Fluffy Egg & Cheese Muffins

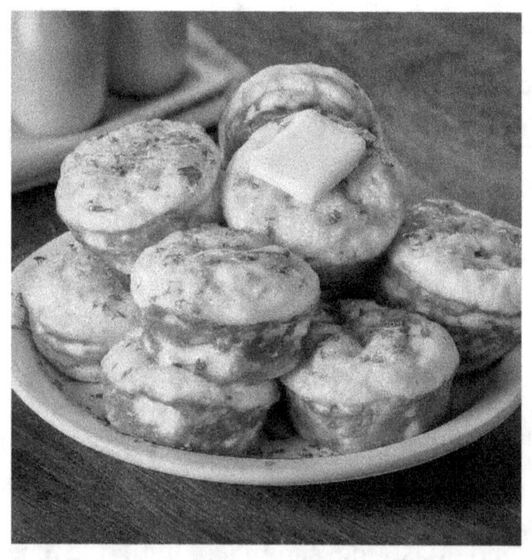

Preparation Time: 15 minutes

Cooking Time: 25 minutes

Ingredients:

- 12 eggs, pasture-raised

- 1 cup heavy cream

- 1 cup shredded cheddar cheese

- 1/2 tsp salt

Instructions:

1. Preheat your oven to 350°F (175°C).

2. In a large bowl, whisk together the eggs, heavy cream, cheddar cheese, and salt until well combined.

3. Grease a 12-cup muffin tin with butter or oil.

4. Evenly distribute the egg mixture into the muffin cups, filling them about 3/4 full.

5. Bake for 20-25 minutes, or until the muffins are set and lightly golden on top.

6. Allow the muffins to cool for 5 minutes before removing them from the tin.

Nutritional Value (per muffin):

- Calories: 204

- Fat: 18g

- Protein: 12g

- Carbohydrates: 1g

3. Carnivore Quiche

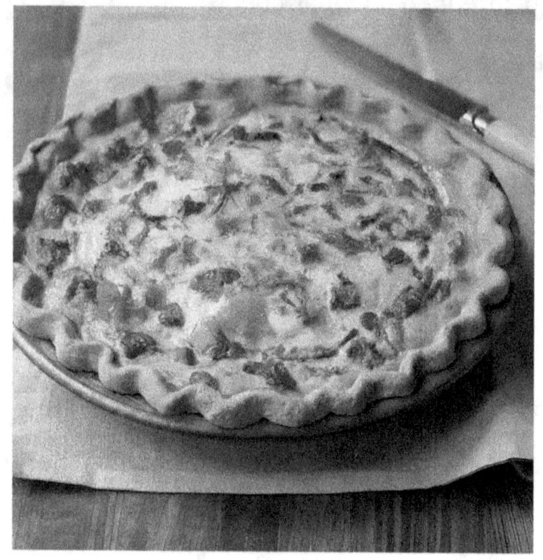

Preparation Time: 20 minutes

Cooking Time: 40 minutes

Ingredients:

- 1 1/4 cups powdered pork rinds

- 1 1/4 cups freshly grated Parmesan cheese or hard

Gouda cheese

- 1 large egg

- Use 1/2 cup of either chicken or beef bone broth.

- Utilize 1 cup of shredded Swiss or Muenster cheese.

- Include 4 ounces of cream cheese.

- 1 tbsp. melted butter

- 1/2 cup diced ham

- 4 large eggs, beaten

- 1/2 tsp sea salt

Instructions:

1. Preheat your oven to 375°F (190°C).

2. In a bowl, mix the powdered pork rinds, Parmesan or Gouda cheese, and 1 egg to form the crust. Press the combined mixture into a pie dish.

3. In a separate bowl, whisk together the broth, shredded cheese, cream cheese, melted butter, diced ham, beaten eggs, and salt.

4. Pour the egg mixture into the prepared crust.

5. Bake for 35-40 minutes, or until the quiche is set and the crust is golden brown.

6. Allow the quiche to cool for 5-10 minutes before slicing and serving.

Nutritional Value (per slice):

- Calories: 320

- Fat: 25g

- Protein: 20g

- Carbohydrates: 3g

4. Carnivore Breakfast Burrito

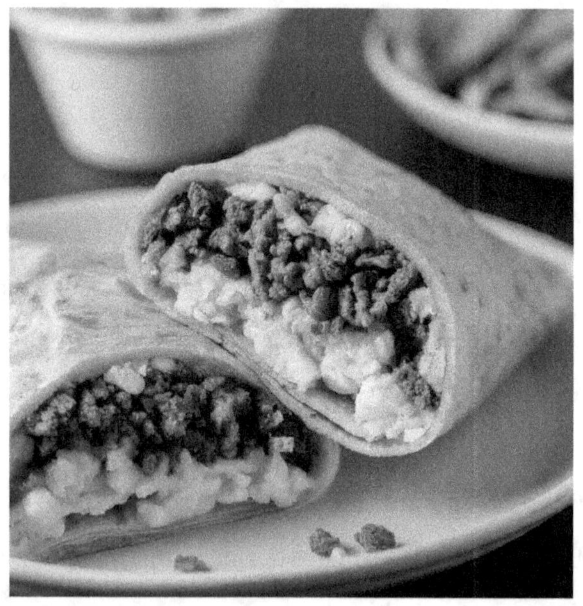

Preparation Time: 15 minutes

Cooking Time: 20 minutes

Ingredients:

- 4 eggs, pasture-raised

- 1/2 lb ground beef

- 2 tbsp. butter

- 1/4 cup shredded cheddar cheese

- 2 large lettuce leaves (for wrapping)

Instructions:

1. In a skillet, cook the ground beef over medium-high heat until browned and cooked through, about 5-7 minutes. Drain any excess fat.

2. In a separate skillet, melt the butter over medium heat. Crack the eggs into the skillet and scramble them until cooked through about 3-5 minutes.

3. Warm the lettuce leaves in the microwave for 30 seconds to make them more pliable.

4. Divide the scrambled eggs and ground beef evenly between the two lettuce leaves. Top each with 2 tbsp of shredded cheddar cheese.

5. Fold the lettuce leaves around the filling to create a burrito-like wrap.

Nutritional Value (per burrito):

- Calories: 380

- Fat: 27g

- Protein: 30g

- Carbohydrates: 2g

5. Carnivore Breakfast Skillet

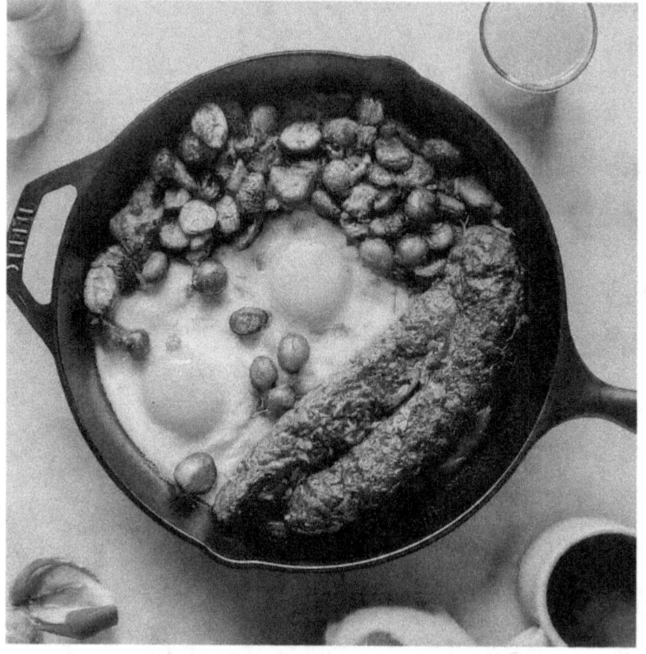

Preparation Time: 10 minutes

Cooking Time: 20 minutes

Ingredients:

- 1 lb. ground pork sausage

- 6 eggs, pasture-raised

- 1/2 cup shredded cheddar cheese

- 2 tbsp. butter

- 1/4 tsp salt

- 1/4 tsp black pepper

Instructions:

1. In a large skillet, cook the ground pork sausage over medium-high heat until browned and cooked through, about 7-10 minutes. Drain any excess fat.

2. Reduce the heat to medium and add the butter to the skillet. Crack the eggs directly into the skillet and scramble them, stirring frequently, until they are cooked to your desired doneness, about 3-5 minutes.

3. Sprinkle the shredded cheddar cheese over the egg and sausage mixture and let it melt for about 1-2 minutes.

4. Season with salt and pepper.

5. Serve the carnivore breakfast skillet hot.

Nutritional Value (per serving):

- Calories: 420

- Fat: 34g

- Protein: 26g

- Carbohydrates: 1g

6. Carnivore Breakfast Meatballs

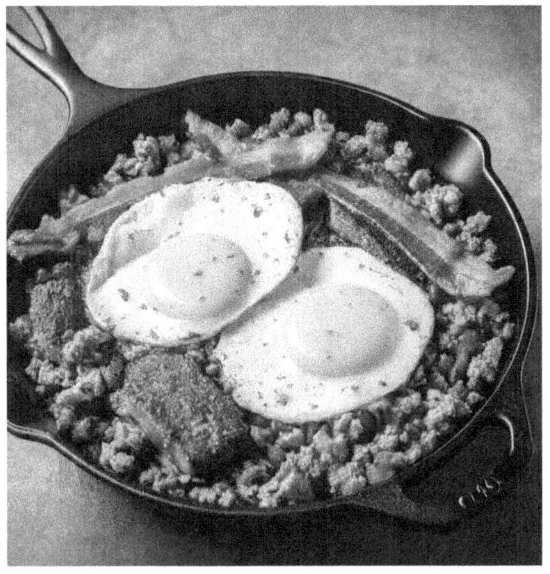

Preparation Time: 15 minutes

Cooking Time: 20 minutes

Ingredients:

- 1 lb. ground beef

- 4 eggs, pasture-raised

- 1/4 cup grated Parmesan cheese

- 1/4 tsp salt

- 1/4 tsp black pepper

- 2 tbsp. butter

Instructions:

1. Preheat your oven to 400°F (200°C).

2. In a large bowl, mix together the ground beef, 2 of the eggs, Parmesan cheese, salt, and pepper until well combined.

3. Roll the mixture into 12 equal-sized meatballs and place them on a baking sheet lined with parchment paper.

4. Bake the meatballs for 15-20 minutes, or until they are cooked through and no longer pink in the center.

5. In a skillet, melt the butter over medium heat. Crack the remaining 2 eggs into the skillet and fry them to your desired doneness.

6. Serve the carnivore breakfast meatballs with the fried eggs.

Nutritional Value (per serving):

- Calories: 350

- Fat: 25g

- Protein: 30g

- Carbohydrates: 1g

7. Carnivore Breakfast Sausage Patties

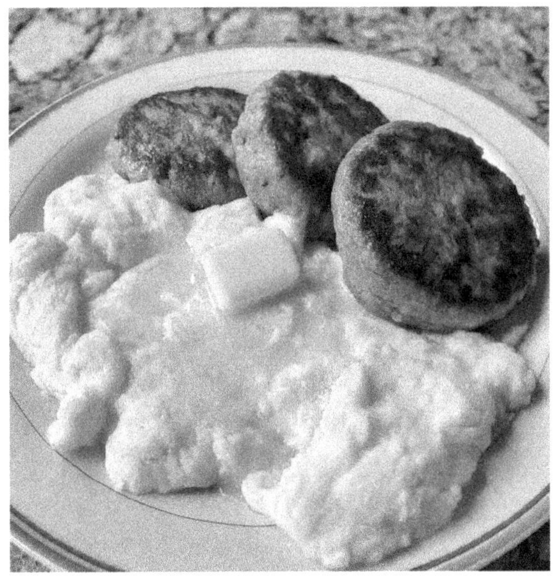

Preparation Time: 10 minutes

Cooking Time: 15 minutes

Ingredients:

- 1 lb. ground pork
- 1 tsp salt
- 1/2 tsp black pepper
- 1/2 tsp dried sage
- 1/4 tsp ground fennel (optional)
- 2 tbsp. butter

Instructions:

1. In a large bowl, mix together the ground pork, salt, black pepper, dried sage, and ground fennel (if using) until well combined.

2. Divide the mixture into 8 equal-sized patties, about 1/2 inch thick.

3. In a sizable skillet, melt the butter over medium-high heat.

4. Cook the sausage patties for 3-4 minutes per side, or until they are cooked through and no longer pink in the center.

5. Serve the carnivore breakfast sausage patties hot.

Nutritional Value (per patty):

- Calories: 180

- Fat: 15g

- Protein: 12g

- Carbohydrates: 0g

8. Carnivore Breakfast Tacos

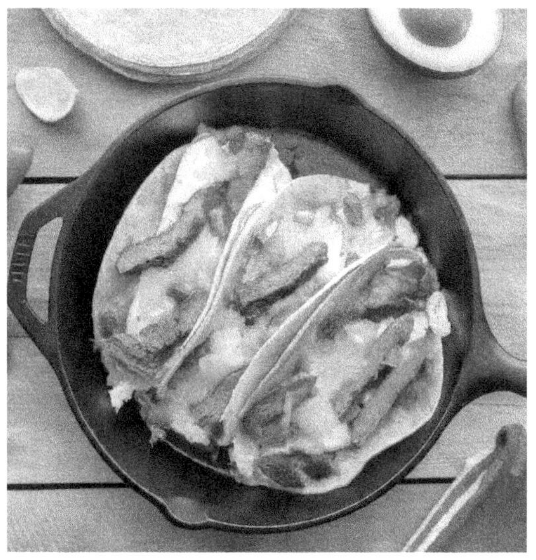

Preparation Time: 15 minutes

Cooking Time: 20 minutes

Ingredients:

- 6 eggs, pasture-raised

- 1/2 lb. ground beef

- 1/4 cup shredded cheddar cheese

- 2 tbsp. butter

- 4 large lettuce leaves (for taco shells)

Instructions:

1. In a skillet, cook the ground beef over medium-high heat until browned and cooked through, about 5-7 minutes. Drain any excess fat.

2. In a separate skillet, melt the butter over medium heat. Crack the eggs into the skillet and scramble them until cooked through, about 3-5 minutes.

3. Warm the lettuce leaves in the microwave for 30 seconds to make them more pliable.

4. Divide the scrambled eggs and ground beef evenly between the four lettuce leaves.

5. Top each taco with 1 tbsp of shredded cheddar cheese.

Nutritional Value (per taco):

- Calories: 260

- Fat: 18g

- Protein: 22g

- Carbohydrates: 2g

9. Carnivore Breakfast Salmon Roll-Ups

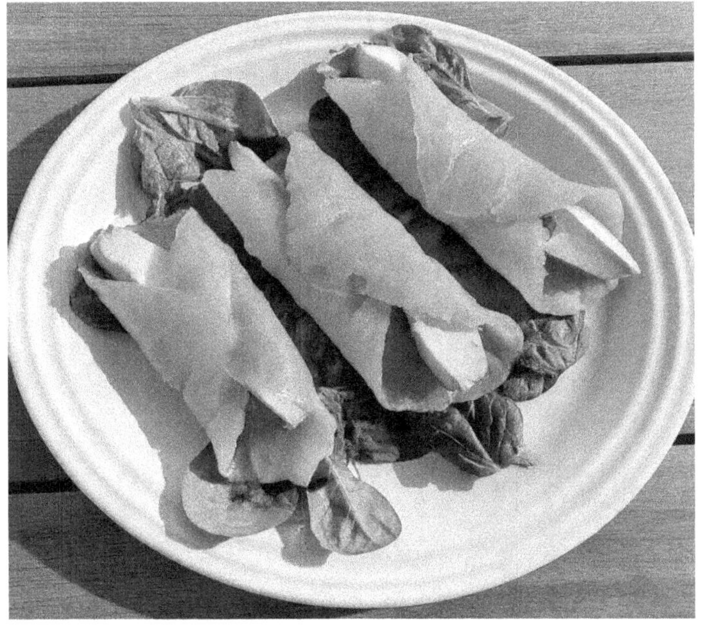

Preparation Time: 10 minutes

Cooking Time: 0 minutes

Ingredients:

- 4 oz. smoked salmon slices

- 2 tbsp. cream cheese

- Chopped fresh dill for garnish (optional)

Instructions:

1. Arrange the smoked salmon slices on a sanitized surface.

2. Spread a thin layer of cream cheese onto each slice.

3. Roll up the salmon slices with the cream cheese inside.

4. Garnish with chopped fresh dill if desired.

5. Savor these delightful carnivore breakfast salmon roll-ups.

Nutritional Value (per roll-up):

- Calories: 90

- Fat: 6g

- Protein: 7g

- Carbohydrates: 0g

10. Carnivore Breakfast Steak and Eggs

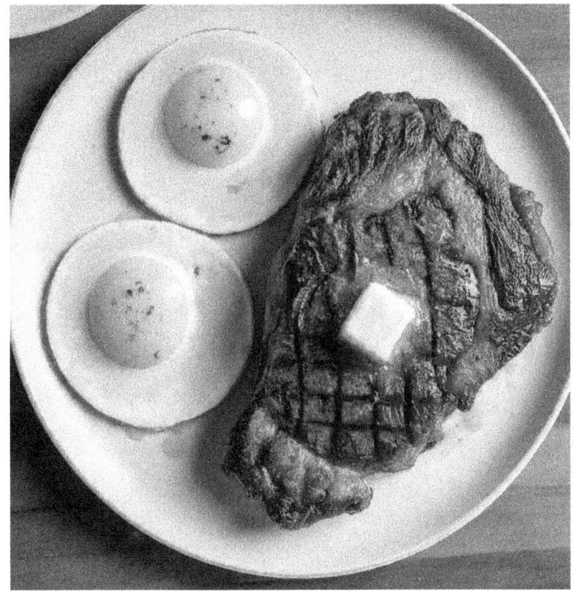

Preparation Time: 5 minutes

Cooking Time: 15 minutes

Ingredients:

- 8 oz. ribeye steak

- 3 eggs, pasture-raised

- 1 tbsp. butter

- Salt and pepper to taste

Instructions:

1. Season the ribeye steak with salt and pepper.

2. In a skillet, melt the butter over medium-high heat.

3. Cook the steak for 3-5 minutes per side, or until it reaches your desired doneness.

4. In a separate skillet, fry the eggs to your desired doneness.

5. Serve the carnivore breakfast steak and eggs hot, with the steak and eggs side by side.

Nutritional Value (per serving):

- Calories: 450

- Fat: 32g

- Protein: 40g

- Carbohydrates: 0g

CHAPTER 3: Carnivore Diet Poultry

11. Carnivore Roasted Chicken

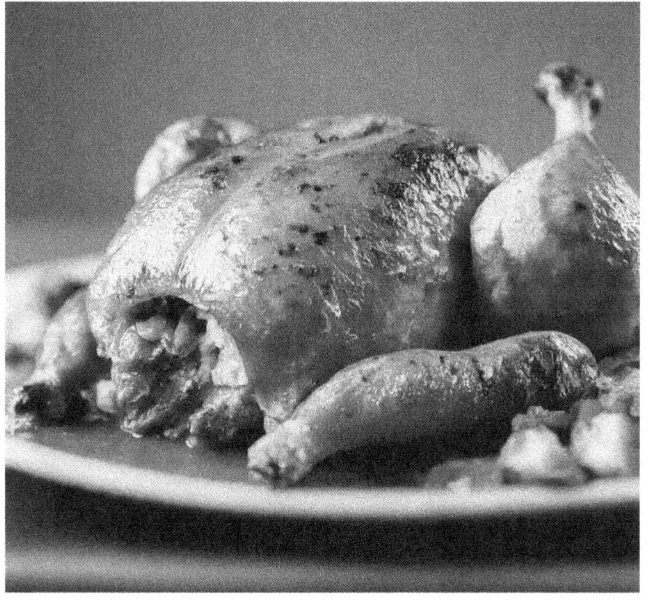

Preparation Time: 15 minutes

Cooking Time: 1 hour 15 minutes

Ingredients:

- 1 whole chicken (4-5 lbs.)

- 2 tbsp. butter, melted

- 1 tsp salt

- 1/2 tsp black pepper

Instructions:

1. Preheat your oven to 425°F (220°C).

2. Dry the chicken with paper towels and then place it into a roasting pan.

3. Brush the chicken all over with the melted butter and season it evenly with the salt and pepper.

4. Roast the chicken for 1 hour and 15 minutes, or until the internal temperature reaches 165°F (75°C) in the thickest part of the thigh.

5. Allow the chicken to rest for 10 minutes before carving and serving.

Nutritional Value (per serving):

- Calories: 450

- Fat: 30g

- Protein: 50g

- Carbohydrates: 0g

12. Carnivore Chicken Thighs with Crispy Skin

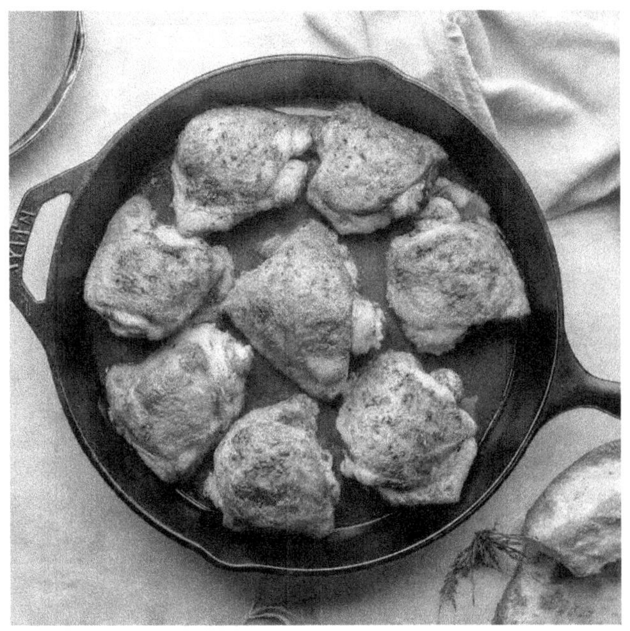

Preparation Time: 10 minutes

Cooking Time: 35 minutes

Ingredients:

- 8 bone-in, skin-on chicken thighs

- 2 tbsp. avocado oil

- 1 tsp salt

- 1/2 tsp black pepper

Instructions:

1. Preheat your oven to 425°F (220°C).

2. Pat the chicken thighs dry with paper towels and season them evenly with the salt and pepper.

3. Heat the avocado oil in a large, oven-safe skillet over medium-high heat.

4. Add the chicken thighs, skin-side down, and cook for 8-10 minutes, or until the skin is crispy and golden brown.

5. Turn over the chicken

6. Roast for 20-25 minutes, or until the chicken is cooked through and the internal temperature reaches 165°F (75°C).

7. Allow the chicken to rest for 5 minutes before serving.

Nutritional Value (per serving):

- Calories: 380

- Fat: 28g

- Protein: 35g

- Carbohydrates: 0g

13. Carnivore Chicken Salad

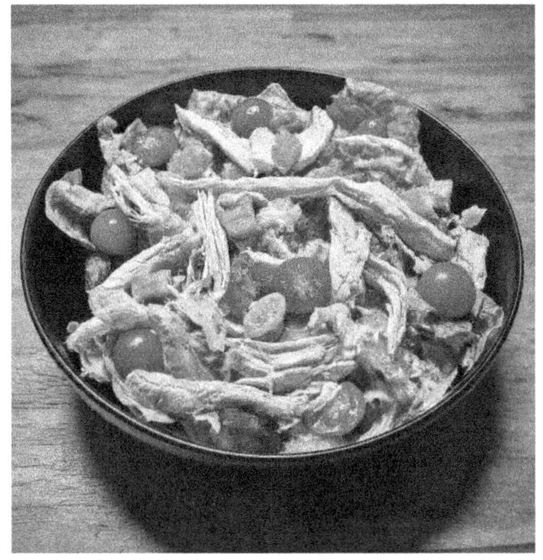

Preparation Time: 15 minutes

Cooking Time: 0 minutes

Ingredients:

- 2 cups cooked, shredded chicken

- 1/2 cup mayonnaise

- 2 tbsp. Dijon mustard

- 1/4 cup diced celery

- 2 tbsp. chopped fresh parsley

- 1 tsp lemon juice

- 1/4 tsp salt

- 1/4 tsp black pepper

Instructions:

1. In a large bowl, combine the shredded chicken, mayonnaise, Dijon mustard, diced celery, chopped parsley, lemon juice, salt, and black pepper.

2. Thoroughly blend until the ingredients are evenly spread throughout.

3. Serve the carnivore chicken salad on its own, or use it as a filling for lettuce wraps or on top of a bed of greens.

Nutritional Value (per serving):

- Calories: 320

- Fat: 25g

- Protein: 25g

- Carbohydrates: 2g

14. Carnivore Chicken Nuggets

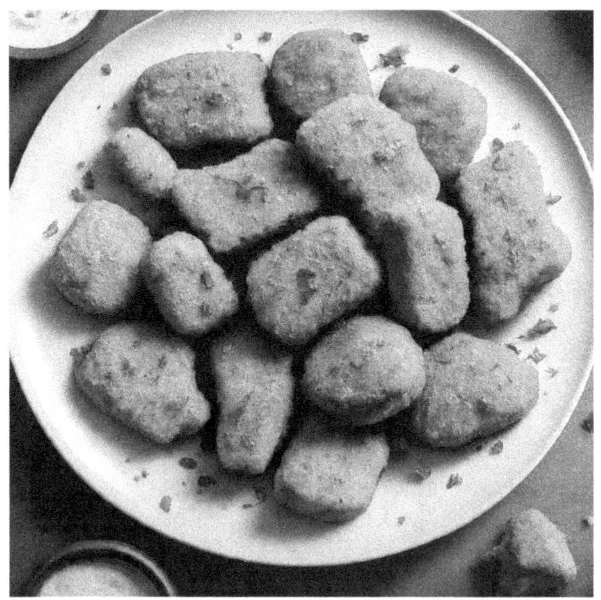

Preparation Time: 20 minutes

Cooking Time: 20 minutes

Ingredients:

- 1 lb boneless, skinless chicken thighs, cut into 1-inch pieces

- 1 cup pork rinds, crushed into a fine powder

- 1/2 cup grated Parmesan cheese

- 1 tsp garlic powder

- 1 tsp onion powder

- 1/2 tsp salt

- 1/4 tsp black pepper

- 2 tbsp. avocado oil

Instructions:

1. Preheat your oven to 400°F (200°C).

2. In a large bowl, combine the crushed pork rinds, Parmesan cheese, garlic powder, onion powder, salt, and black pepper.

3. Toss the chicken pieces in the pork rind mixture until they are evenly coated.

4. Arrange the coated chicken nuggets on a baking sheet lined with parchment paper.

5. Drizzle the avocado oil over the chicken nuggets.

6. Bake for 20 minutes, flipping halfway through, until the chicken is cooked through and the coating is crispy.

7. Serve the carnivore chicken nuggets hot.

Nutritional Value (per serving):

- Calories: 280

- Fat: 18g

- Protein: 25g

- Carbohydrates: 2g

15. Carnivore Chicken Wings

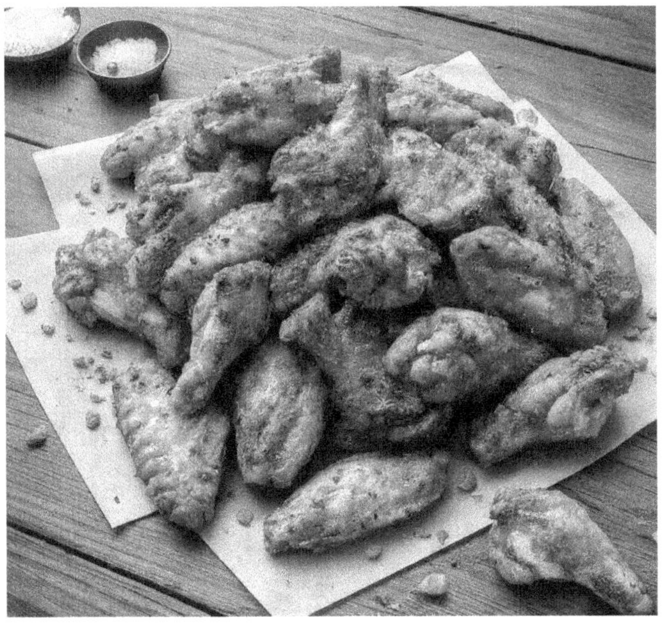

Preparation Time: 10 minutes

Cooking Time: 45 minutes

Ingredients:

- 2 lbs. chicken wings, roomettes and flats separated

- 2 tbsp. baking powder

- 1 tsp salt

- 1/2 tsp black pepper

Instructions:

1. Preheat your oven to 400°F (200°C).

2. Dry the chicken wings with paper towels and place them into a spacious bowl.

3. Sprinkle the baking powder, salt, and black pepper over the wings and toss to coat them evenly.

4. Arrange the wings in a single layer on a baking sheet lined with parchment paper.

5. Bake for 45 minutes, flipping the wings halfway through, until they are crispy and cooked through.

6. Serve the carnivore chicken wings hot.

Nutritional Value (per serving):

- Calories: 350

- Fat: 22g

- Protein: 40g

- Carbohydrates: 0g

16. Carnivore Chicken Meatballs

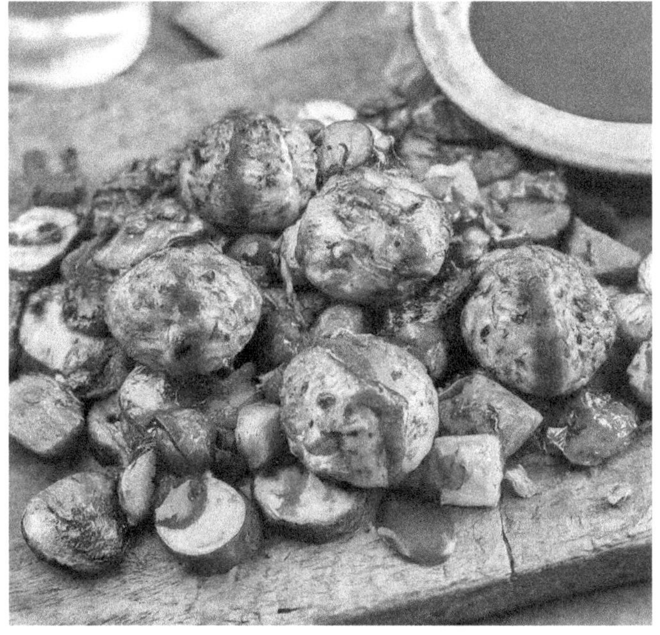

Preparation Time: 15 minutes

Cooking Time: 20 minutes

Ingredients:

- 1 lb. ground chicken

- 2 eggs, beaten

- 1/4 cup grated Parmesan cheese

- 1 tsp dried oregano

- 1/2 tsp salt

- 1/4 tsp black pepper

- 2 tbsp. avocado oil

Instructions:

1. Preheat your oven to 400°F (200°C).

2. In a large bowl, combine the ground chicken, beaten eggs, Parmesan cheese, dried oregano, salt, and black pepper. Thoroughly combine the ingredients until they are evenly spread.

3. Then, shape the mixture into meatballs about 1 inch in size and arrange them on a baking sheet lined with parchment paper.

4. Drizzle the avocado oil over the meatballs.

5. Bake for 20 minutes, or until the meatballs are cooked through and no longer pink in the center.

6. Serve the carnivore chicken meatballs hot.

- Calories: 260

- Fat: 16g

- Protein: 25g

- Carbohydrates: 1g

17. Carnivore Chicken Parmesan

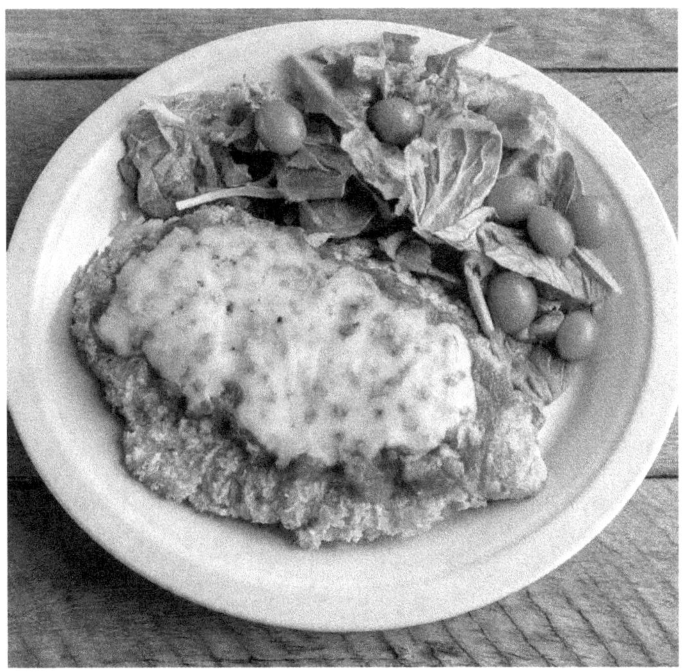

Preparation Time: 20 minutes

Cooking Time: 30 minutes

 Ingredients:

- 4 boneless, skinless chicken breasts

- 1 cup grated Parmesan cheese

- 1/2 cup heavy cream

- 1 tsp dried basil

- 1/2 tsp garlic powder

- 1/4 tsp salt

- 1/4 tsp black pepper

- 2 tbsp. butter

 Instructions:

1. Preheat your oven to 400°F (200°C).

2. Pound the chicken breasts between two sheets of parchment paper to an even thickness of about 1/2 inch.

3. In a shallow bowl, mix together the Parmesan cheese, heavy cream, dried basil, garlic powder, salt, and black pepper.

4. Dip the chicken breasts in the Parmesan mixture, coating both sides.

5. Melt the butter in a large, oven-safe skillet over medium-high heat.

6. Add the coated chicken breasts to the skillet and cook for 2-3 minutes per side, or until the cheese is lightly browned.

7. Transfer the skillet to the preheated oven and bake for 20-25 minutes, or until the chicken is cooked through and the cheese is melted and bubbly.

8. Serve the carnivore chicken parmesan hot.

Nutritional Value (per serving):

- Calories: 420

- Fat: 28g

- Protein: 40g

- Carbohydrates: 2g

18. Carnivore Chicken Fajitas

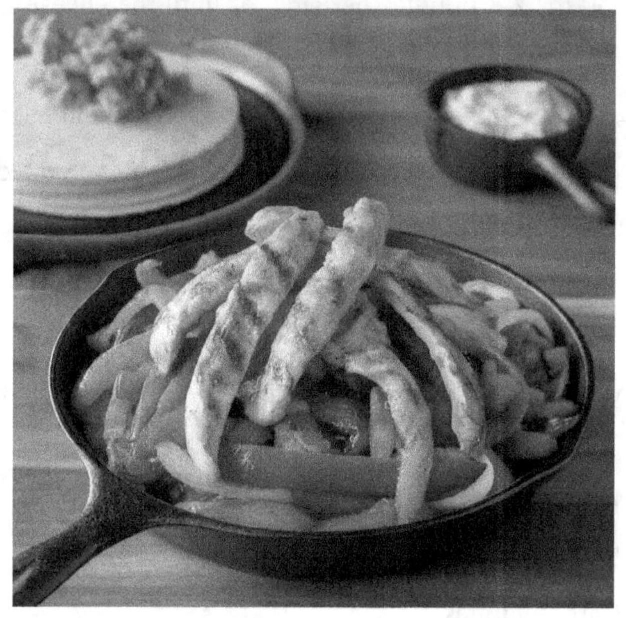

Preparation Time: 15 minutes

Cooking Time: 20 minutes

Ingredients:

- 1 lb. boneless, skinless chicken thighs, sliced into strips

- 1 red bell pepper, sliced

- 1 green bell pepper, sliced

- 1 onion, sliced

- 2 tbsp avocado oil

- 1 tsp chili powder

- 1 tsp cumin

- 1/2 tsp garlic powder

- 1/2 tsp salt

- 1/4 tsp black pepper

- Lettuce leaves for serving

Instructions:

1. In a large skillet, heat the avocado oil over medium-high heat.

2. Add the sliced chicken, bell peppers, and onion to the skillet. Season with the chili powder, cumin, garlic powder, salt, and black pepper.

3. Sauté the mixture, stirring occasionally, for 15-20 minutes, or until the chicken is cooked through and the vegetables are tender.

4. Serve the carnivore chicken fajitas in lettuce leaves.

Nutritional Value (per serving):

- Calories: 320

- Fat: 20g

- Protein: 35g

- Carbohydrates: 8g

19. Carnivore Chicken Soup

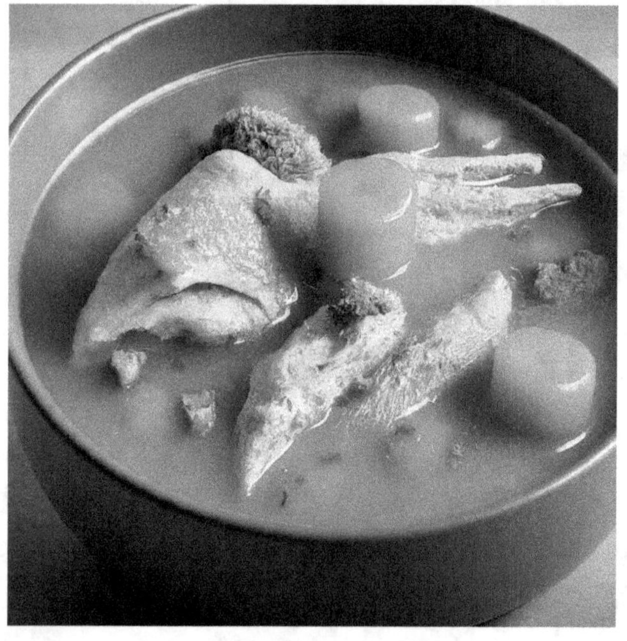

Preparation Time: 20 minutes

Cooking Time: 1 hour

Ingredients:

- 1 whole chicken (4-5 lbs.), cut into 8 pieces

- 8 cups chicken bone broth

- 2 celery stalks, diced

- 2 carrots, diced

- 1 onion, diced

- 2 cloves garlic, minced

- 1 tsp dried thyme

- 1 tsp dried parsley

- 1 tsp salt

- 1/2 tsp black pepper

Instructions:

1. In a large pot, combine the chicken pieces, chicken bone broth, celery, carrots, onion, garlic, dried thyme, dried parsley, salt, and black pepper.

2. Bring the mixture to a boil over high heat, then reduce the heat to medium-low and simmer for 1 hour, or until the chicken is cooked through and the vegetables are tender.

3. Remove the chicken pieces from the pot and shred the meat off the bones. Discard the bones.

4. Return the shredded chicken to the pot and stir to combine.

5. Serve the carnivore chicken soup hot.

Nutritional Value (per serving):

- Calories: 380

- Fat: 22g

- Protein: 40g

- Carbohydrates: 6g

20. Carnivore Chicken Liver Pâté

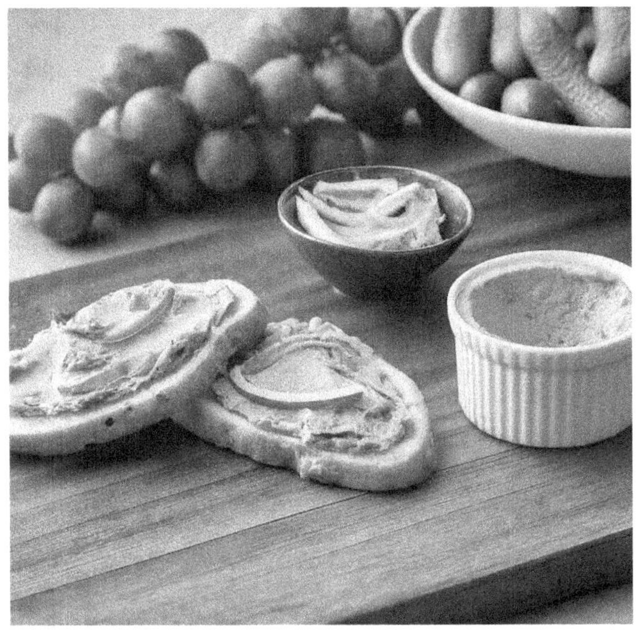

Preparation Time: 15 minutes

Cooking Time: 30 minutes

Ingredients:

- 1 lb. chicken livers, trimmed

- 1/2 cup butter, softened

- 2 tbsp. heavy cream

- 1 tsp salt

- 1/2 tsp black pepper

- 1/4 tsp ground nutmeg

Instructions:

1. In a large skillet, cook the chicken livers over medium-high heat for 5-7 minutes, or until they are cooked through and no longer pink. Allow to cool slightly.

2. In a food processor, combine the cooked chicken livers, softened butter, heavy cream, salt, black pepper, and ground nutmeg. Blend until smooth and creamy.

3. Transfer the pâté to a serving dish or ramekins and refrigerate for at least 2 hours, or until firm.

4. Serve the carnivore chicken liver pâté chilled, with additional butter or tallow for dipping.

Nutritional Value (per serving):

- Calories: 280

- Fat: 22g

- Protein: 18g

- Carbohydrates: 1g

CHAPTER 4: Carnivore Diet Beef

21. Carnivore Ribeye Steak

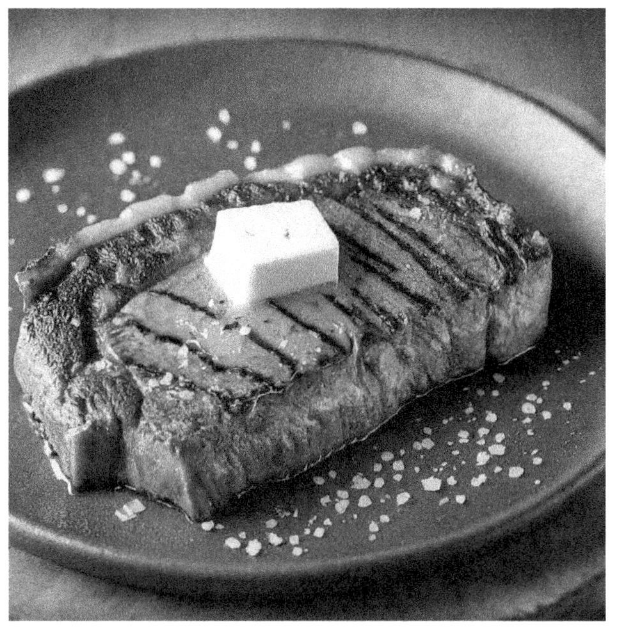

Preparation Time: 5 minutes

Cooking Time: 10-15 minutes

Ingredients:

- 2 (8 oz.) ribeye steaks, about 1-inch thick

- 1 tbsp. avocado oil

- 1 tsp salt

- 1/2 tsp black pepper

Instructions:

1. Pat the ribeye steaks dry with paper towels and let them come to room temperature, about 30 minutes.

2. Preheat a cast-iron skillet or grill pan over high heat.

3. Rub the steaks all over with the avocado oil and season generously with the salt and pepper.

4. Sear the steaks for 4-5 minutes per side, or until they reach your desired level of doneness.

5. Transfer the steaks to a cutting board and let them rest for 5-10 minutes before slicing and serving.

Nutritional Value (per serving):

- Calories: 450

- Fat: 35g

- Protein: 40g

- Carbohydrates: 0g

22. Carnivore Beef Burgers

Preparation Time: 10 minutes

Cooking Time: 10-12 minutes

Ingredients:

- 1 lb. ground beef

- 1 tsp salt

- 1/2 tsp black pepper

- 2 tbsp. butter or tallow for cooking

Instructions:

1. in a large bowl, gently mix together the ground beef, salt, and black pepper until just combined, being careful not to overmix.

2. Divide the mixture into 4 equal portions and shape them into patties, about 1/2 inch thick.

3. In a large skillet or on a grill, melt the butter or tallow over medium-high heat.

4. Cook the beef patties for 5-6 minutes per side, or until they reach your desired level of doneness.

5. Serve the carnivore beef burgers hot, with your favorite carnivore-friendly toppings.

Nutritional Value (per serving):

- Calories: 320

- Fat: 24g

- Protein: 28g

- Carbohydrates: 0g

23. Carnivore Beef Chili

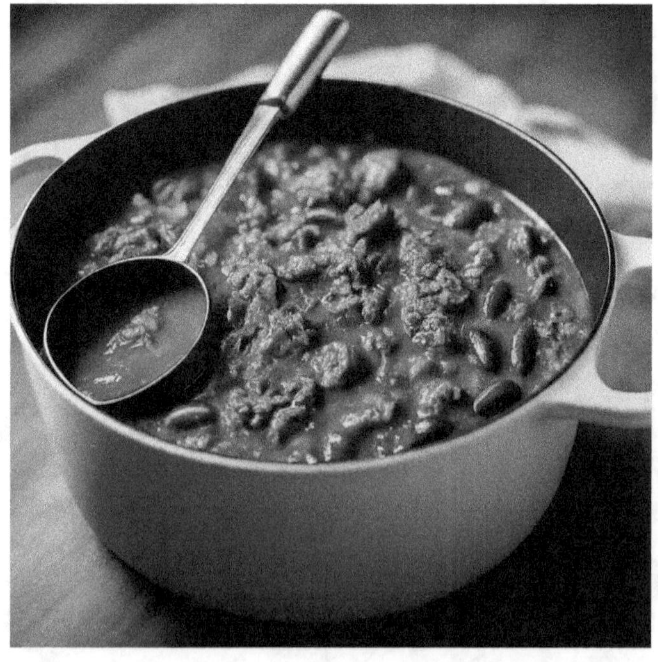

Preparation Time: 15 minutes

Cooking Time: 1 hour

Ingredients:

- 2 lbs. ground beef

- 1 onion, diced

- 3 cloves garlic, minced

- 2 tbsp. chili powder

- 1 tsp ground cumin

- 1 tsp dried oregano

- 1 tsp salt

- 1/2 tsp black pepper

- 1 cup beef bone broth

Instructions:

1. In a large pot or Dutch oven, cook the ground beef over medium-high heat, breaking it up with a wooden spoon, until browned and cooked through, about 8-10 minutes.

2. Add the diced onion and minced garlic to the pot and sauté for 3-4 minutes, until the onion is translucent.

3. Stir in the chili powder, cumin, dried oregano, salt, and black pepper. Cook for 2-3 minutes until the spices are toasted.

4. Pour in the beef bone broth and bring the mixture to a simmer.

5. Reduce the heat to low and let the carnivore beef chili simmer for 45 minutes to 1 hour, stirring occasionally, until the flavors have melded and the chili has thickened.

6. Serve hot.

Nutritional Value (per serving):
- Calories: 380
- Fat: 24g
- Protein: 35g
- Carbohydrates: 4g

24. Carnivore Beef Meatballs

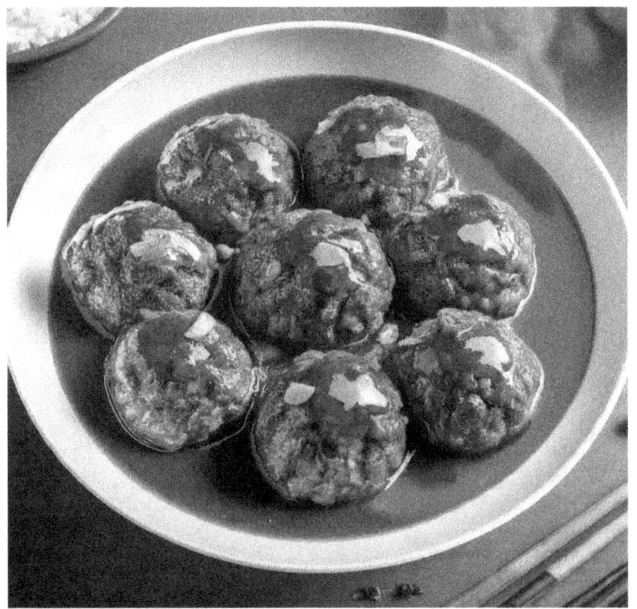

Preparation Time: 15 minutes

Cooking Time: 20 minutes

Ingredients:

- 1 lb. ground beef

- 2 eggs, beaten

- 1/2 cup grated Parmesan cheese

- 1 tsp dried oregano

- 1 tsp salt

- 1/2 tsp black pepper

- 2 tbsp. avocado oil

Instructions:

1. Preheat your oven to 400°F (200°C).

2. In a large bowl, combine the ground beef, beaten eggs, Parmesan cheese, dried oregano, salt, and black pepper. Thoroughly blend until all the ingredients are evenly dispersed.

3. Shape the mixture into 1-inch meatballs and arrange them on a baking sheet covered with parchment paper.

4. Drizzle the avocado oil over the meatballs.

5. Bake for 20 minutes, or until the meatballs are cooked through and no longer pink in the center.

6. Serve the carnivore beef meatballs hot.

Nutritional Value (per serving):

- Calories: 280

- Fat: 18g

- Protein: 25g

- Carbohydrates: 1g

25. Carnivore Beef Stroganoff

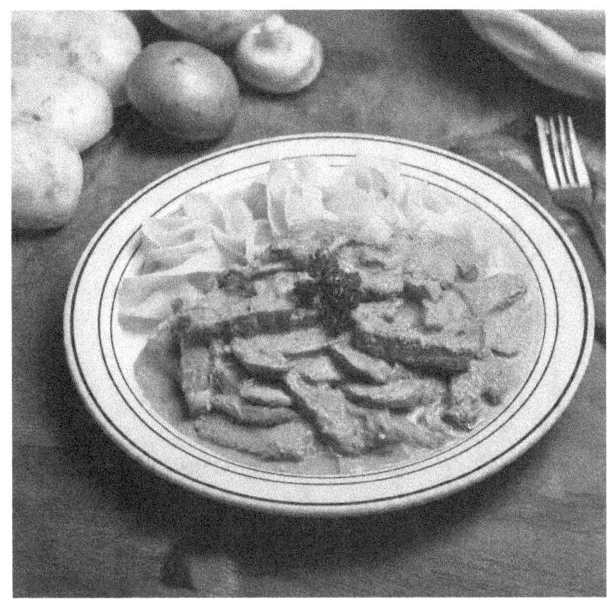

Preparation Time: 20 minutes

Cooking Time: 30 minutes

Ingredients:

- 1 lb. beef tenderloin or sirloin, cut into 1-inch cubes

- 2 tbsp. butter

- 1 onion, diced

- 8 oz. mushrooms, sliced

- 1 cup beef bone broth

- 1/2 cup heavy cream

- 1 tsp Dijon mustard

- 1/2 tsp salt

- 1/4 tsp black pepper

Instructions:

1. In a sizable skillet, melt the butter on medium-high heat.

2. Add the beef cubes and sear them on all sides, about 2-3 minutes per side. Take out the beef from the skillet and place it aside.

3. Add the diced onion to the skillet and sauté for 3-4 minutes, until translucent.

4. Add the sliced mushrooms to the skillet and cook for an additional 5 minutes.

5. Pour in the beef bone broth and scrape up any browned bits from the bottom of the skillet.

6. Stir in the heavy cream, Dijon mustard, salt, and black pepper. Bring the mixture to a simmer.

7. Return the seared beef cubes to the skillet and let the carnivore beef stroganoff simmer for 15-20 minutes, or until the beef is tender and the sauce has thickened.

8. Serve hot.

Nutritional Value (per serving):

- Calories: 420

- Fat: 30g

- Protein: 35g

- Carbohydrates: 4g

26. Carnivore Beef Brisket

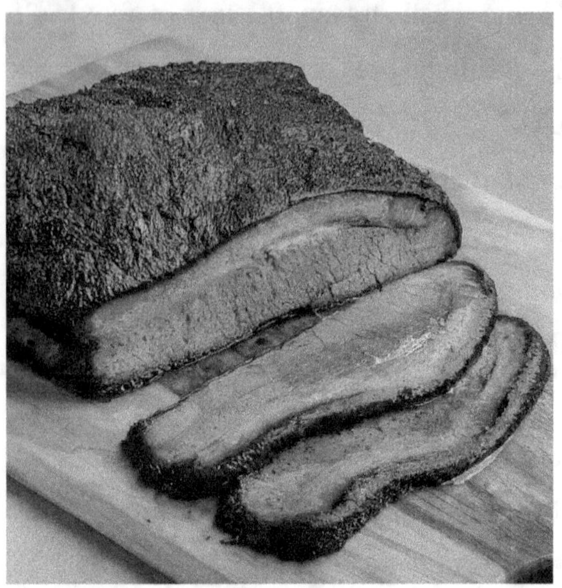

Preparation Time: 15 minutes

Cooking Time: 8-10 hours

Ingredients:

- 4 lb. beef brisket

- 2 tbsp. salt

- 1 tbsp. black pepper

- 1 tbsp. garlic powder

- 1 tbsp. onion powder

- 1/4 cup beef tallow or avocado oil

Instructions:

1. Preheat your oven to 275°F (135°C).

2. Pat the beef brisket dry with paper towels and season it all over with the salt, black pepper, garlic powder, and onion powder.

3. Heat the beef tallow or avocado oil in a large, oven-safe Dutch oven or roasting pan over medium-high heat.

4. Sear the brisket on all sides until a nice crust forms, about 2-3 minutes per side.

5. Cover the Dutch oven or roasting pan with a tight-fitting lid or aluminum foil.

6. Transfer the pan to the preheated oven and roast the brisket for 8-10 hours, or until it is fork-tender.

7. Remove the brisket from the oven and let it rest for 15-20 minutes before slicing and serving.

Nutritional Value (per serving):

- Calories: 450

- Fat: 30g

- Protein: 45g

- Carbohydrates: 0g

27. Carnivore Beef Stew

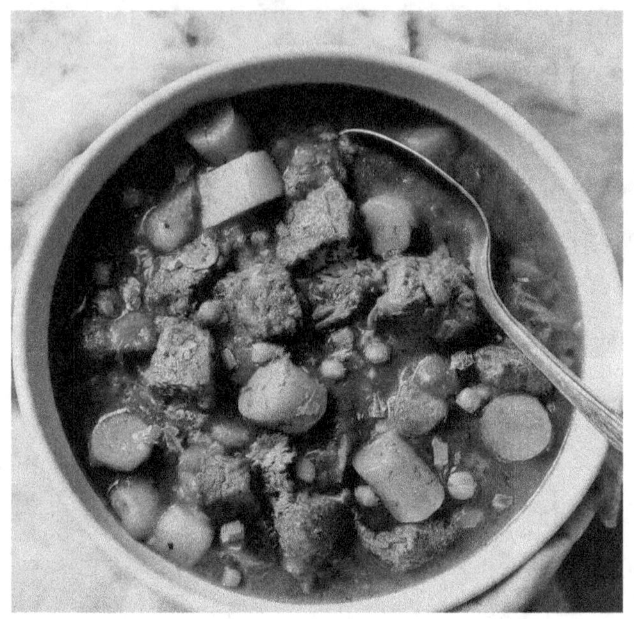

Preparation Time: 20 minutes

Cooking Time: 2 hours

Ingredients:

- 2 lbs. beef chuck, cut into 1-inch cubes

- 1 onion, diced

- 3 carrots, peeled and diced

- 3 celery stalks, diced

- 4 cups beef bone broth

- 1 tsp dried thyme

- 1 tsp salt

- 1/2 tsp black pepper

- 2 tbsp. butter

Instructions:

1. In a large pot or Dutch oven, melt the butter over medium-high heat.

2. Add the beef cubes and sear them on all sides, about 2-3 minutes per side. Take the beef out of the pot and place it aside.

3. Add the diced onion, carrots, and celery to the pot and sauté for 5-7 minutes, until the vegetables are starting to soften.

4. Pour in the beef bone broth and add the seared beef cubes back to the pot. Stir in the dried thyme, salt, and black pepper.

5. Bring the mixture to a boil, then reduce the heat to low, cover the pot, and let the carnivore beef stew simmer for 1 1/2 to 2 hours, or until the beef is very tender.

6. Serve hot.

Nutritional Value (per serving):

- Calories: 380

- Fat: 22g

- Protein: 40g

- Carbohydrates: 8g

28. Carnivore Beef Liver Pâté

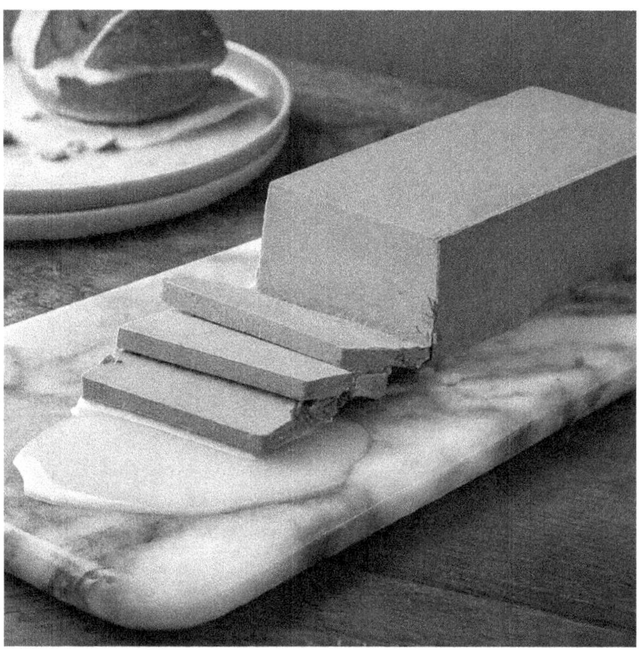

Preparation Time: 15 minutes

Cooking Time: 15 minutes

Ingredients:

- 1 lb. beef liver, trimmed

- 1/2 cup butter, softened

- 2 tbsp. heavy cream

- 1 tsp salt

- 1/2 tsp black pepper

- 1/4 tsp ground nutmeg

Instructions:

1. in a large skillet, cook the beef liver over medium-high heat for 5-7 minutes, or until it is cooked through and no longer pink. Allow to cool slightly.

2. In a food processor, combine the cooked beef liver, softened butter, heavy cream, salt, black pepper, and ground nutmeg. Blend until smooth and creamy.

3. Transfer the pâté to a serving dish or ramekins and refrigerate for at least 2 hours, or until firm.

4. Serve the carnivore beef liver pâté chilled, with additional butter or tallow for dipping.

Nutritional Value (per serving):

- Calories: 300

- Fat: 24g

- Protein: 20g

- Carbohydrates: 1g

29. Carnivore Beef Tartare

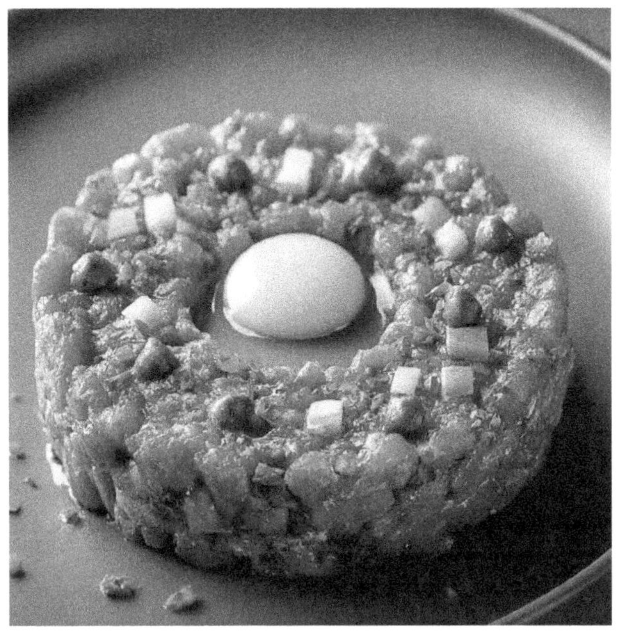

Preparation Time: 15 minutes

Cooking Time: 0 minutes

Ingredients:

- 1 lb. grass-fed beef tenderloin, finely chopped

- 2 egg yolks

- 2 tbsp. Dijon mustard

- 1 tbsp. capers, drained and chopped

- 1 tbsp. finely chopped shallot

- 1 tsp Worcestershire sauce

- 1 tsp lemon juice

- 1/2 tsp salt

- 1/4 tsp black pepper

Instructions:

1. In a large bowl, gently mix together the chopped beef tenderloin, egg yolks, Dijon mustard, capers, chopped shallot, Worcestershire sauce, lemon juice, salt, and black pepper until well combined.

2. Divide the carnivore beef tartare mixture into 4 equal portions and shape them into small mounds or patties.

3. Serve the beef tartare chilled, with additional Dijon mustard, capers, or other carnivore-friendly garnishes, if desired.

Nutritional Value (per serving):

- Calories: 280

- Fat: 18g

- Protein: 30g

- Carbohydrates: 2g

30. Carnivore Beef Jerky

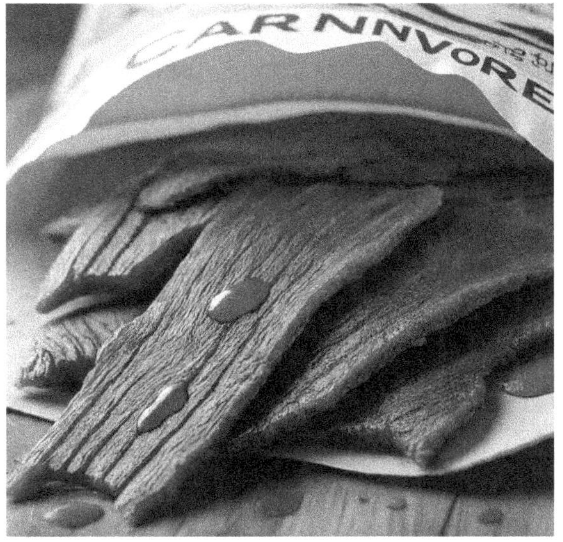

Preparation Time: 20 minutes

Cooking Time: 4-6 hours

Ingredients:

- 2 lbs beef flank steak or top round, sliced into 1/4-inch thick strips

- 2 tbsp salt

- 1 tbsp. black pepper

- 1 tsp garlic powder

- 1 tsp onion powder

Instructions:

1. Pat the beef strips dry with paper towels and place them in a large bowl.

2. In a small bowl, mix together the salt, black pepper, garlic powder, and onion powder.

3. Sprinkle the spice mixture over the beef strips and toss to coat them evenly.

4. Arrange the seasoned beef strips in a single layer on dehydrator trays or a baking sheet lined with a wire rack.

5. Dehydrate the beef jerky in a dehydrator at 155°F (68°C) for 4-6 hours, or until the jerky is dry and leathery, but still pliable.

6. Alternatively, you can bake the jerky in a preheated 175°F (80°C) oven for 4-6 hours, flipping the strips halfway through.

7. Store the carnivore beef jerky in an airtight container at room temperature for up to 2 weeks.

Nutritional Value (per serving):

- Calories: 120

- Fat: 4g

- Protein: 18g

- Carbohydrates: 0g

CHAPTER 4: Carnivore Diet Pork and Lamb

31. Carnivore Pork Chops

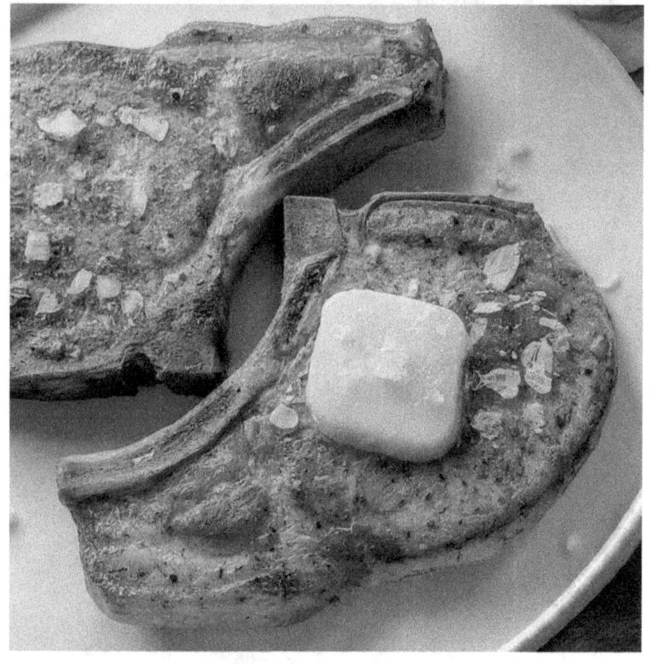

Preparation Time: 5 minutes

Cooking Time: 12-15 minutes

Ingredients:

- 4 (8 oz.) bone-in pork chops, about 1-inch thick

- 1 tbsp. avocado oil

- 1 tsp salt

- 1/2 tsp black pepper

Instructions:

1. Pat the pork chops dry with paper towels and let them come to room temperature, about 30 minutes.

2. Preheat a cast-iron skillet or grill pan over medium-high heat.

3. Rub the pork chops all over with the avocado oil and season generously with the salt and pepper.

4. Cook the pork chops for 5-6 minutes on each side, or until they reach an internal temperature of 145°F (63°C) through.

5. Transfer the pork chops to a cutting board and let them rest for 5 minutes before serving.

Nutritional Value (per serving):

- Calories: 380

- Fat: 22g

- Protein: 45g

- Carbohydrates: 0g

32. Carnivore Pork Belly

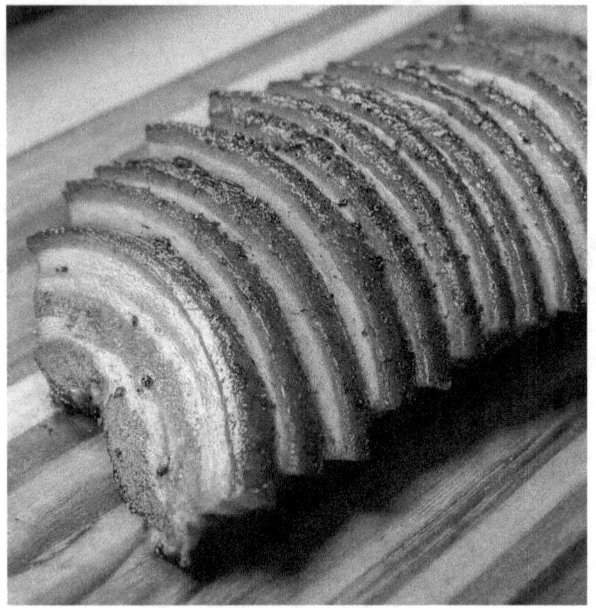

Preparation Time: 10 minutes

Cooking Time: 2-3 hours

Ingredients:

- 2 lbs. pork belly, skin on

- 1 tbsp. salt

- 1 tsp black pepper

- 1 tbsp. baking soda

Instructions:

1. Preheat your oven to 300°F (150°C).

2. Pat the pork belly dry with paper towels and score the skin in a crosshatch pattern, being careful not to cut too deep into the meat.

3. Rub the salt, black pepper, and baking soda all over the pork belly, including the skin.

4. Place the pork belly, skin-side up, on a wire rack set over a baking sheet.

5. Roast the pork belly for 2-3 hours, or until the skin is crispy and the meat is tender.

6. Let the pork belly rest for 10 minutes before slicing and serving.

Nutritional Value (per serving):

- Calories: 450

- Fat: 35g

- Protein: 35g

- Carbohydrates: 0g

33. Carnivore Pork Sausage

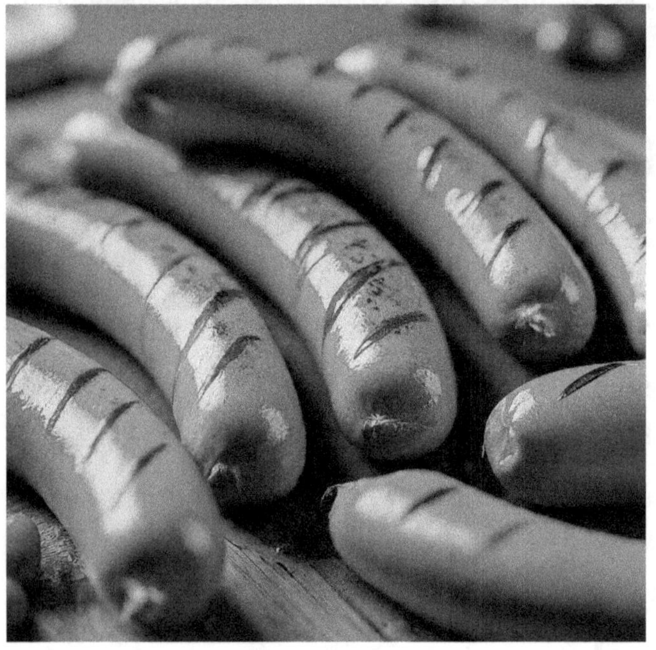

Preparation Time: 15 minutes

Cooking Time: 15-20 minutes

Ingredients:

- 2 lbs. ground pork

- 1 tbsp. salt

- 1 tsp black pepper

- 1 tsp dried sage

- 1/2 tsp ground fennel (optional)

- 2 tbsp. butter or tallow for cooking

Instructions:

1. In a large bowl, mix together the ground pork, salt, black pepper, dried sage, and ground fennel (if using) until well combined.

2. Divide the mixture into 8 equal-sized patties, about 1/2 inch thick.

3. In a large skillet, melt the butter or tallow over medium-high heat.

4. Cook the pork sausage patties for 7-8 minutes per side, or until they are cooked through and no longer pink in the center.

5. Serve the carnivore pork sausage hot.

Nutritional Value (per serving):

- Calories: 320

- Fat: 25g

- Protein: 22g

- Carbohydrates: 0g

34. Carnivore Lamb Chops

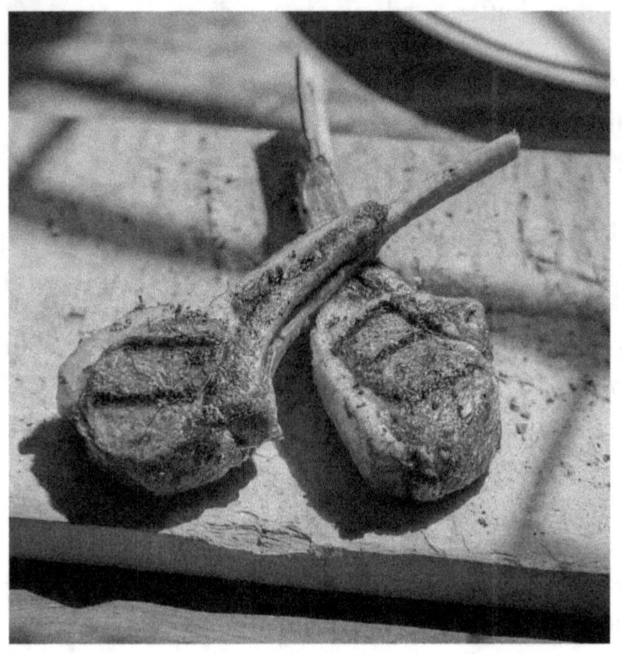

Preparation Time: 5 minutes

Cooking Time: 8-10 minutes

Ingredients:

- 4 (8 oz.) lamb chops, about 1-inch thick

- 1 tbsp. avocado oil

- 1 tsp salt

- 1/2 tsp black pepper

Instructions:

1. Pat the lamb chops dry with paper towels and let them come to room temperature, about 30 minutes.

2. Preheat a cast-iron skillet or grill pan over medium-high heat.

3. Rub the lamb chops all over with the avocado oil and season generously with the salt and pepper.

4. Sear the lamb chops for 4-5 minutes per side, or until they reach an internal temperature of 130°F (55°C) for medium-rare.

5. Transfer the lamb chops to a cutting board and let them rest for 5 minutes before serving.

Nutritional Value (per serving):

- Calories: 380

- Fat: 25g

- Protein: 40g

- Carbohydrates: 0g

35. Carnivore Lamb Meatballs

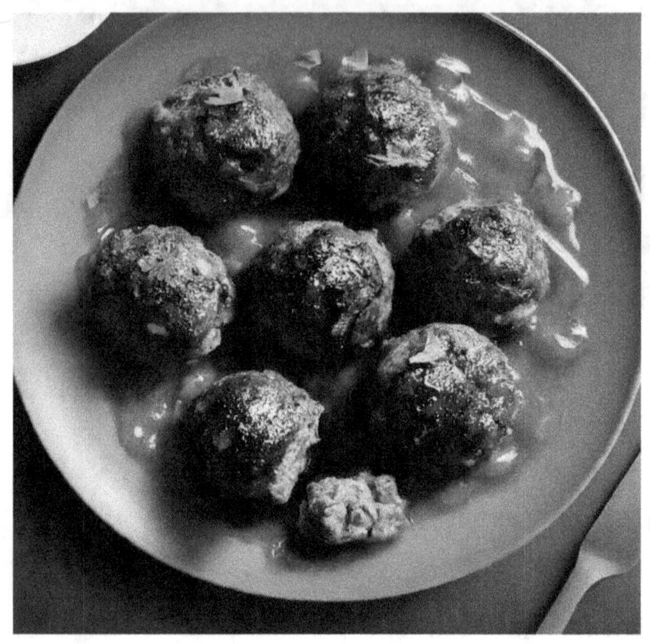

Preparation Time: 15 minutes

Cooking Time: 20 minutes

Ingredients:

- 1 lb. ground lamb

- 2 eggs, beaten

- 1/2 cup grated Parmesan cheese

- 1 tsp dried oregano

- 1 tsp salt

- 1/2 tsp black pepper

- 2 tbsp. avocado oil

Instructions:

1. Preheat your oven to 400°F (200°C).

2. In a large bowl, combine the ground lamb, beaten eggs, Parmesan cheese, dried oregano, salt, and black pepper. Thoroughly blend until all the ingredients are evenly incorporated.

3. Shape the mixture into meatballs about 1 inch in size and arrange them on a baking sheet covered with parchment paper.

4. Drizzle the avocado oil over the meatballs.

5. Bake for 20 minutes, or until the meatballs are cooked through and no longer pink in the center.

6. Serve the carnivore lamb meatballs hot.

Nutritional Value (per serving):

- Calories: 300

- Fat: 20g

- Protein: 28g

- Carbohydrates: 1g

36. Carnivore Lamb Stew

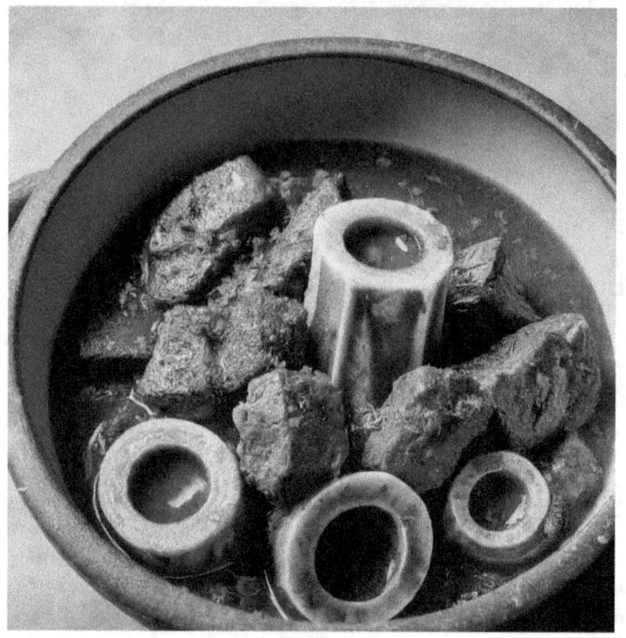

Preparation Time: 20 minutes

Cooking Time: 2 hours

Ingredients:

- 2 pounds of lamb stew meat, chopped into 1-inch pieces.

- 1 onion, diced

- 3 carrots, peeled and diced

- 3 celery stalks, diced

- 4 cups beef bone broth

- 1 tsp dried thyme

- 1 tsp salt

- 1/2 tsp black pepper

- 2 tbsp. butter

Instructions:

1. In a large pot or Dutch oven, melt the butter over medium-high heat.

2. Add the lamb cubes and sear them on all sides, about 2-3 minutes per side. Remove the lamb from the pot and set aside.

3. Add the diced onion, carrots, and celery to the pot and sauté for 5-7 minutes, until the vegetables are starting to soften.

4. Pour in the beef bone broth and add the seared lamb cubes back to the pot. Stir in the dried thyme, salt, and black pepper.

5. Bring the mixture to a boil, then reduce the heat to low, cover the pot, and let the carnivore lamb stew simmer for 1 1/2 to 2 hours, or until the lamb is very tender.

6. Serve hot.

Nutritional Value (per serving):

- Calories: 400

- Fat: 25g

- Protein: 40g

- Carbohydrates: 6g

37. Carnivore Pork Rinds

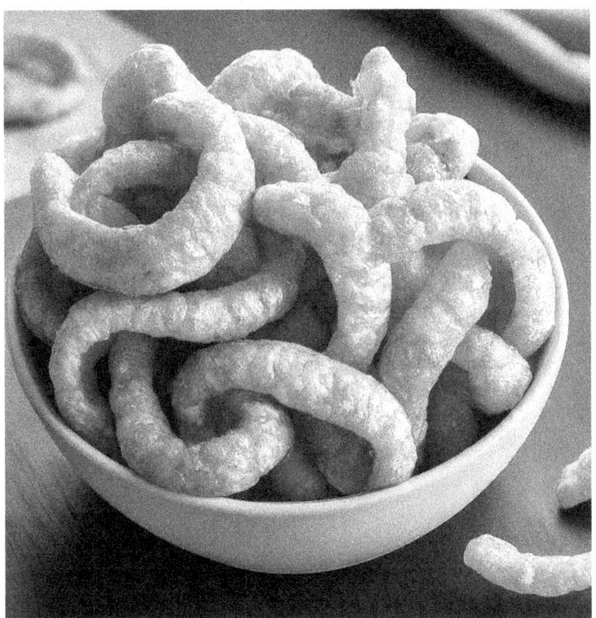

Preparation Time: 10 minutes

Cooking Time: 15-20 minutes

Ingredients:

- 1 lb. pork skin, with fat attached

- 1 tsp salt

Instructions:

1. Preheat your oven to 400°F (200°C).

2. Pat the pork skin dry with paper towels and cut it into 1-inch pieces.

3. Arrange the pork skin pieces in a single layer on a baking sheet.

4. Sprinkle the salt evenly over the pork skin.

5. Bake for 15-20 minutes, or until the pork rinds are puffed and golden brown.

6. Allow the carnivore pork rinds to cool completely before serving.

Nutritional Value (per serving):

- Calories: 150

- Fat: 10g

- Protein: 15g

- Carbohydrates: 0g

38. Carnivore Pork Tenderloin

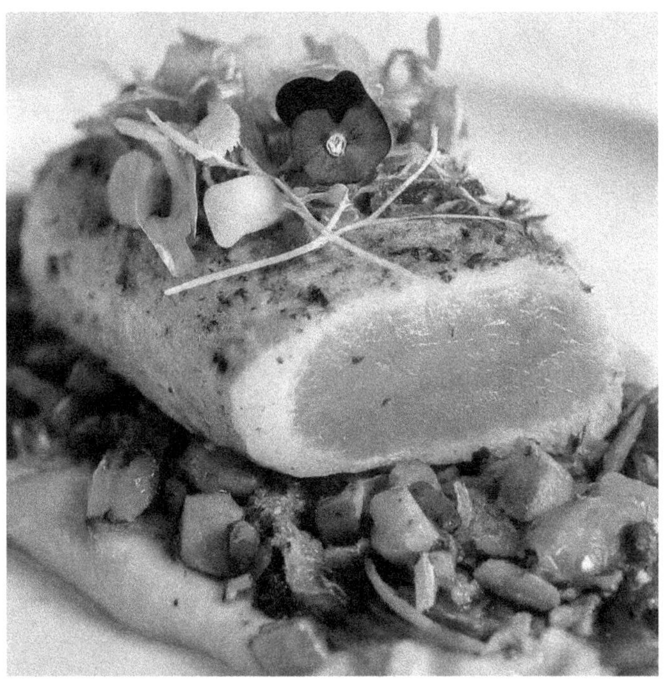

Preparation Time: 10 minutes

Cooking Time: 20-25 minutes

Ingredients:

- 1 lb. pork tenderloin

- 1 tbsp. avocado oil

- 1 tsp salt

- 1/2 tsp black pepper

Instructions:

1. Preheat your oven to 400°F (200°C).

2. Pat the pork tenderloin dry with paper towels and rub it all over with the avocado oil, salt, and black pepper.

3. Place the pork tenderloin on a baking sheet or in a roasting pan.

4. Roast the pork tenderloin for 20-25 minutes, or until it reaches an internal temperature of 145°F (63°C).

5. Allow the pork tenderloin to rest for 5-10 minutes before slicing and serving.

Nutritional Value (per serving):

- Calories: 220

- Fat: 10g

- Protein: 30g

- Carbohydrates: 0g

39. Carnivore Lamb Burgers

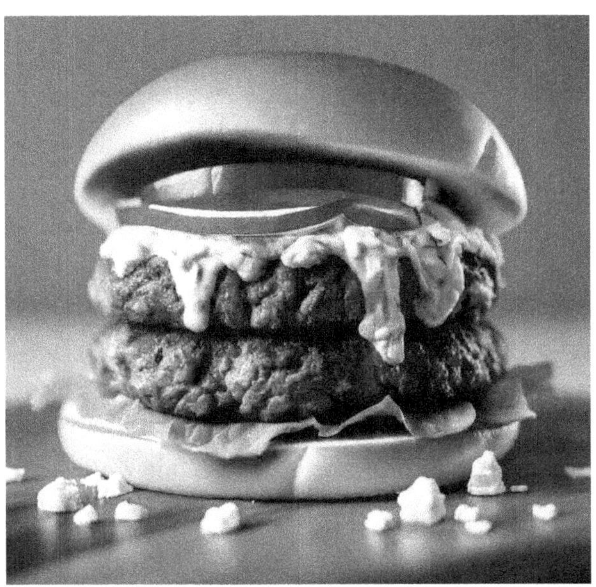

Preparation Time: 10 minutes

Cooking Time: 10-12 minutes

Ingredients:

- 1 lb. ground lamb

- 1 tsp salt

- 1/2 tsp black pepper

- 2 tbsp. butter or tallow for cooking

Instructions:

1. in a large bowl, gently mix together the ground lamb, salt, and black pepper until just combined, being careful not to overmix.

2. Divide the mixture into 4 equal portions and shape them into patties, about 1/2 inch thick.

3. In a large skillet or on a grill, melt the butter or tallow over medium-high heat.

4. Cook the lamb patties for 5-6 minutes per side, or until they reach your desired level of doneness.

5. Serve the carnivore lamb burgers hot, with your favorite carnivore-friendly toppings.

Nutritional Value (per serving):

- Calories: 340

- Fat: 26g

- Protein: 30g

- Carbohydrates: 0g

40. Carnivore Pork Belly Bites

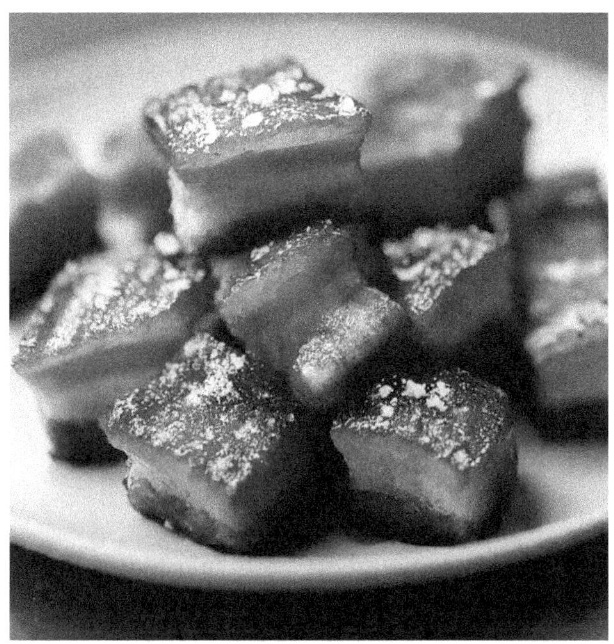

Preparation Time: 10 minutes

Cooking Time: 30-40 minutes

Ingredients:

- 1 pound of pork belly, chopped into 1-inch pieces.

- 1 tbsp. salt

- 1 tsp black pepper

- 1 tbsp. baking soda

Instructions:

1. Preheat your oven to 400°F (200°C).

2. Pat the pork belly cubes dry with paper towels and place them in a large bowl.

3. Sprinkle the salt, black pepper, and baking soda over the pork belly cubes and toss to coat them evenly.

4. Arrange the seasoned pork belly cubes in a single layer on a baking sheet lined with parchment paper.

5. Roast the pork belly bites for 30-40 minutes, or until they are crispy and golden brown.

6. Serve the carnivore pork belly bites hot.

Nutritional Value (per serving):

- Calories: 220

- Fat: 18g

- Protein: 15g

- Carbohydrates: 0g

CHAPTER 5: Carnivore Fish and Seafood

41. Carnivore Grilled Salmon

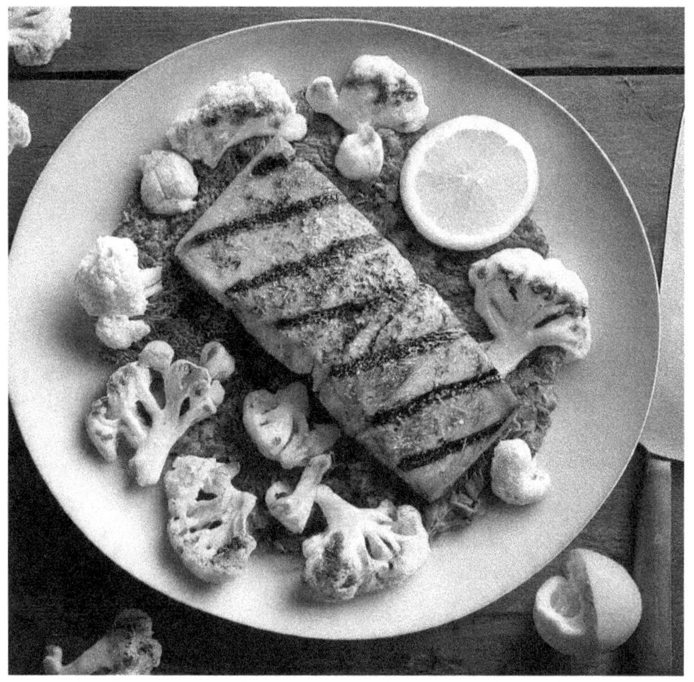

Preparation Time: 5 minutes

Cooking Time: 10-12 minutes

Ingredients:

- 4 (6 Oz) salmon filets

- 1 tbsp. avocado oil

- 1 tsp salt

- 1/2 tsp black pepper

Instructions:

1. Heat your grill or grill pan to medium-high temperature before using it.

2. Pat the salmon filets dry with paper towels and brush them all over with the avocado oil.

3. Season the salmon filets evenly with the salt and black pepper.

4. Grill the salmon for 5-6 minutes per side, or until it flakes easily with a fork and reaches an internal temperature of 145°F (63°C).

5. Serve the carnivore grilled salmon hot.

Nutritional Value (per serving):

- Calories: 320

- Fat: 20g

- Protein: 35g

- Carbohydrates: 0g

42. Carnivore Baked Cod

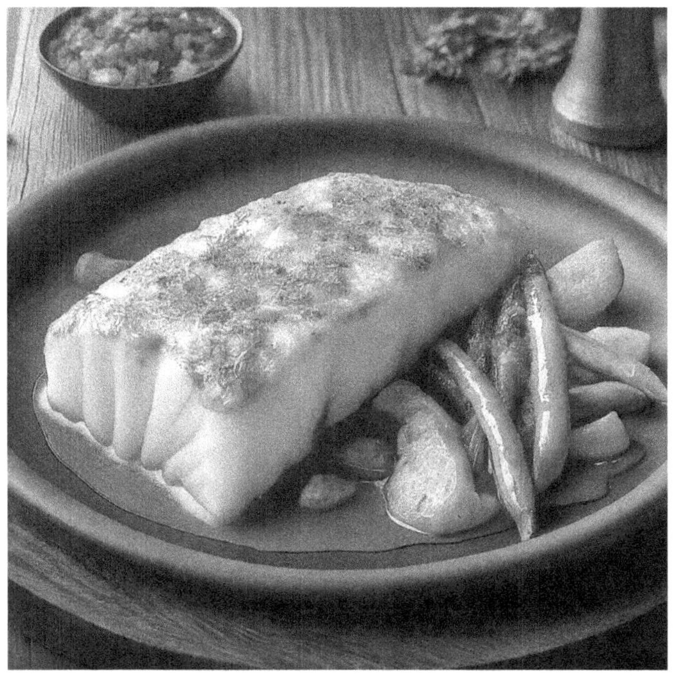

Preparation Time: 5 minutes

Cooking Time: 15-18 minutes

Ingredients:

- 4 (6 Oz) cod filets

- 2 tbsp. butter, melted

- 1 tsp salt

- 1/2 tsp black pepper

Instructions:

1. Preheat your oven to 400°F (200°C).

2. Pat the cod filets dry with paper towels and place them in a baking dish.

3. Brush the cod filets all over with the melted butter and season them evenly with the salt and black pepper.

4. Bake the cod for 15-18 minutes, or until it flakes easily with a fork and reaches an internal temperature of 145°F (63°C).

5. Serve the carnivore-baked cod hot.

Nutritional Value (per serving):

- Calories: 220

- Fat: 10g

- Protein: 30g

- Carbohydrates: 0g

43. Carnivore Shrimp Scampi

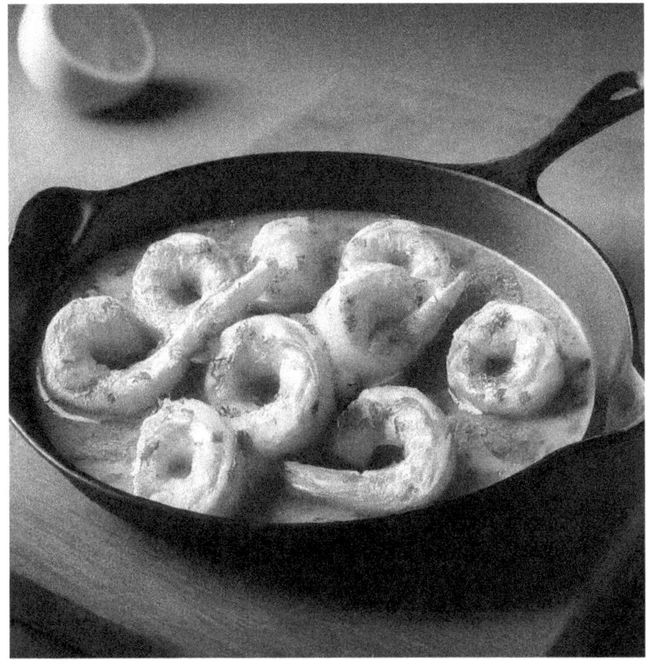

Preparation Time: 10 minutes

Cooking Time: 10 minutes

Ingredients:

- 1 lb. large shrimp, peeled and deveined

- 4 tbsp. butter

- 3 cloves garlic, minced

- 1/4 cup dry white wine (optional)

- 1 tsp lemon juice

- 1/4 tsp red pepper flakes (optional)

- 1 tsp salt

- 1/2 tsp black pepper

Instructions:

1. In a sizable skillet, melt the butter on medium-high heat.

2. Add the minced garlic and sauté for 1 minute, or until fragrant.

3. Add the shrimp to the skillet and cook for 2-3 minutes per side, or until they are pink and opaque.

4. If using, pour in the white wine and let it simmer for 1-2 minutes, allowing the alcohol to cook off.

5. Stir in the lemon juice, red pepper flakes (if using), salt, and black pepper.

6. Serve the carnivore shrimp scampi hot.

Nutritional Value (per serving):

- Calories: 280

- Fat: 18g

- Protein: 25g

- Carbohydrates: 2g

44. Carnivore Seared Scallops

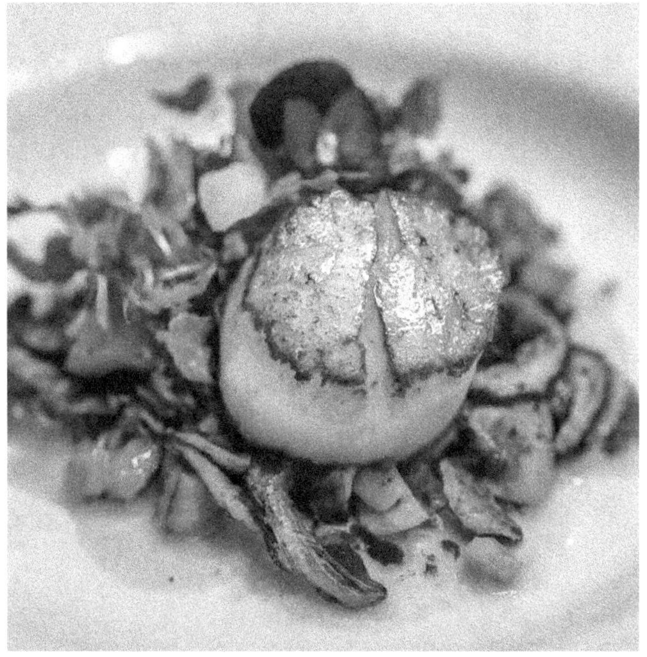

Preparation Time: 5 minutes

Cooking Time: 5-7 minutes

Ingredients:

- 1 lb. sea scallops, patted dry

- 2 tbsp. avocado oil

- 1 tsp salt

- 1/2 tsp black pepper

Instructions:

1. Heat a large skillet or cast-iron pan over high heat.

2. Pat the scallops dry with paper towels and season them evenly with the salt and black pepper.

3. Add the avocado oil to the hot skillet.

4. Carefully add the scallops to the skillet, making sure not to overcrowd them.

5. Sear the scallops for 2-3 minutes per side, or until they are golden brown and cooked through.

6. Serve the carnivore-seared scallops immediately.

Nutritional Value (per serving):

- Calories: 200

- Fat: 10g

- Protein: 25g

- Carbohydrates: 0g

45. Carnivore Crab Cakes

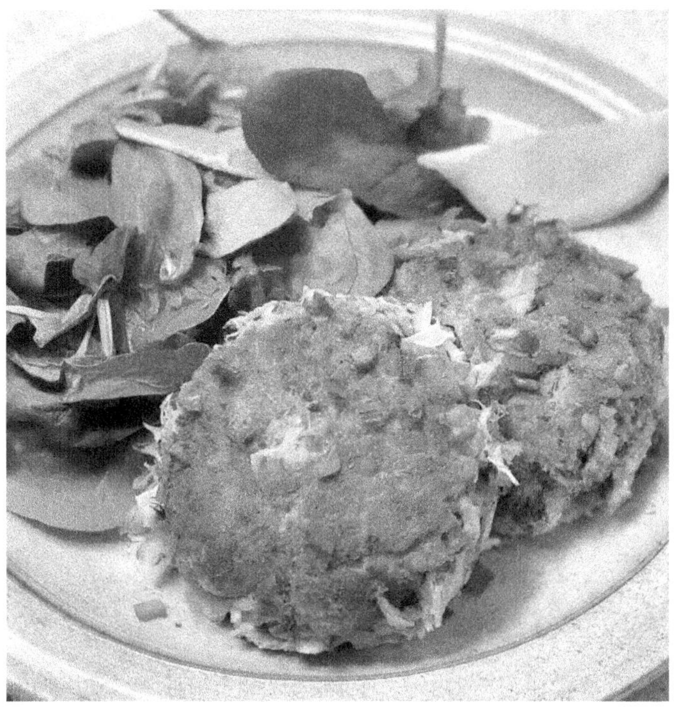

Preparation Time: 15 minutes

Cooking Time: 10-12 minutes

Ingredients:

- 1 lb. lump crabmeat, picked over for shells

- 2 eggs, beaten

- 1/4 cup grated Parmesan cheese

- 2 tbsp. avocado oil

- 1 tsp Dijon mustard

- 1/2 tsp salt

- 1/4 tsp black pepper

Instructions:

1. In a large bowl, gently mix the crabmeat, beaten eggs, Parmesan cheese, Dijon mustard, salt, and black pepper until just combined.

2. Form the mixture into 8 equal-sized crab cakes, about 1/2 inch thick.

3. In a large skillet, heat the avocado oil over medium-high heat.

4. Carefully add the crab cakes to the skillet and cook for 5-6 minutes per side, or until they are golden brown and heated through.

5. Serve the carnivore crab cakes hot.

Nutritional Value (per serving):

- Calories: 240

- Fat: 14g

- Protein: 22g

- Carbohydrates: 2g

46. Carnivore Baked Lobster Tails

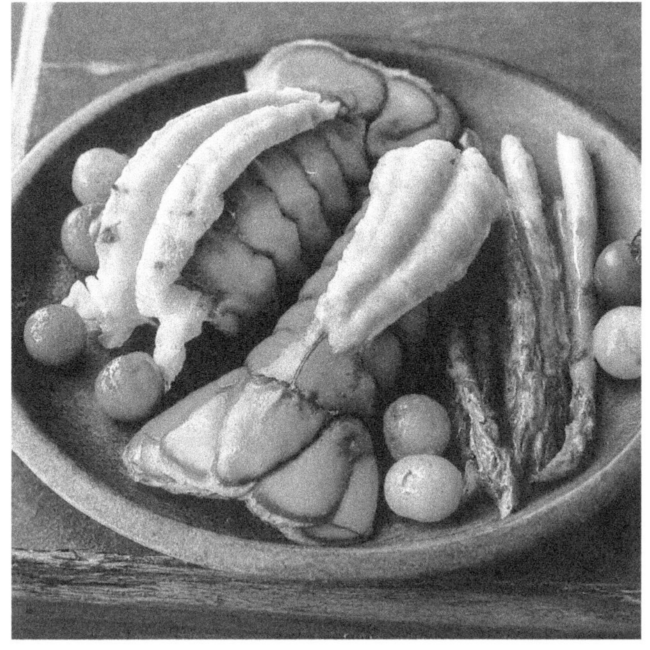

Preparation Time: 10 minutes

Cooking Time: 12-15 minutes

Ingredients:

- 4 (4 Oz) lobster tails

- 2 tbsp butter, melted

- 1 tsp paprika

- 1/2 tsp salt

- 1/4 tsp black pepper

Instructions:

1. Preheat your oven to 400°F (200°C).

2. Using kitchen shears, cut the top shell of the lobster tails lengthwise, being careful not to cut all the way through.

3. Gently pull the meat up and out of the shells, leaving the tail end attached.

4. Place the lobster tails in a baking dish and brush the meat with the melted butter.

5. Sprinkle the paprika, salt, and black pepper evenly over the lobster meat.

6. Bake the lobster tails for 12-15 minutes, or until the meat is opaque and cooked through.

7. Serve the carnivore-baked lobster tails hot.

Nutritional Value (per serving):

- Calories: 180

- Fat: 8g

- Protein: 25g

- Carbohydrates: 0g

47. Carnivore Grilled Tuna Steaks

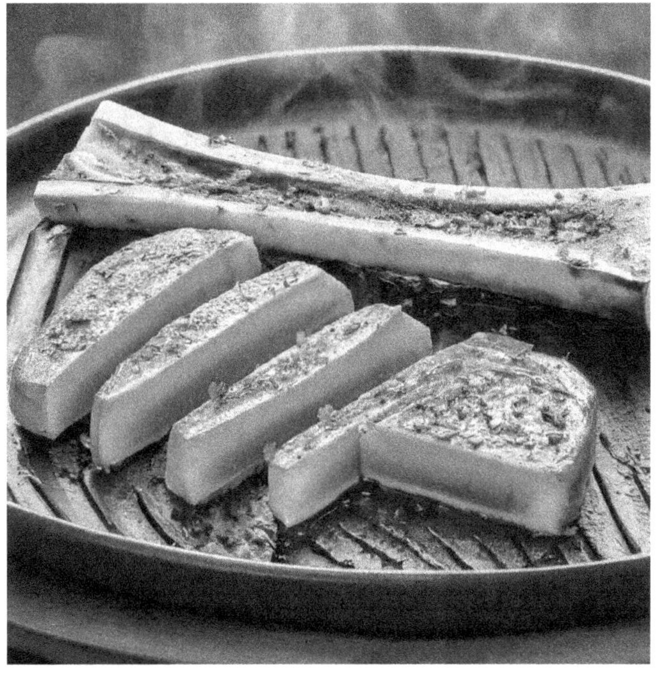

Preparation Time: 5 minutes

Cooking Time: 8-10 minutes

Ingredients:

- 4 (6 Oz) tuna steaks

- 1 tbsp. avocado oil

- 1 tsp salt

- 1/2 tsp black pepper

Instructions:

1. Preheat your grill or grill pan to medium-high heat.

2. Pat the tuna steaks dry with paper towels and brush them all over with the avocado oil.

3. Season the tuna steaks evenly with the salt and black pepper.

4. Grill the tuna for 4-5 minutes per side, or until it reaches your desired level of doneness.

5. Serve the carnivore grilled tuna steaks hot.

Nutritional Value (per serving):

- Calories: 280

- Fat: 12g

- Protein: 40g

- Carbohydrates: 0g

48. Carnivore Seared Ahi Tuna

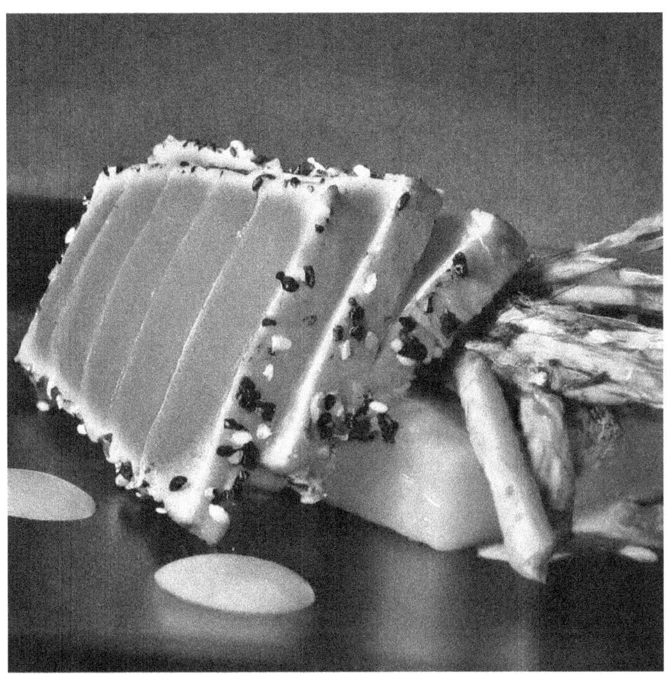

Preparation Time: 5 minutes

Cooking Time: 2-3 minutes

Ingredients:

- 4 (4 Oz) ahi tuna steaks

- 1 tbsp. avocado oil

- 1 tsp salt

- 1/2 tsp black pepper

Instructions:

1. Heat a large skillet or cast-iron pan over high heat.

2. Pat the ahi tuna steaks dry with paper towels and season them evenly with the salt and black pepper.

3. Add the avocado oil to the hot skillet.

4. Carefully add the tuna steaks to the skillet and sear them for 1-2 minutes per side, or until the outside is lightly browned but the center is still rare.

5. Serve the carnivore seared ahi tuna immediately.

Nutritional Value (per serving):

- Calories: 180

- Fat: 8g

- Protein: 25g

- Carbohydrates: 0g

49. Carnivore Baked Halibut

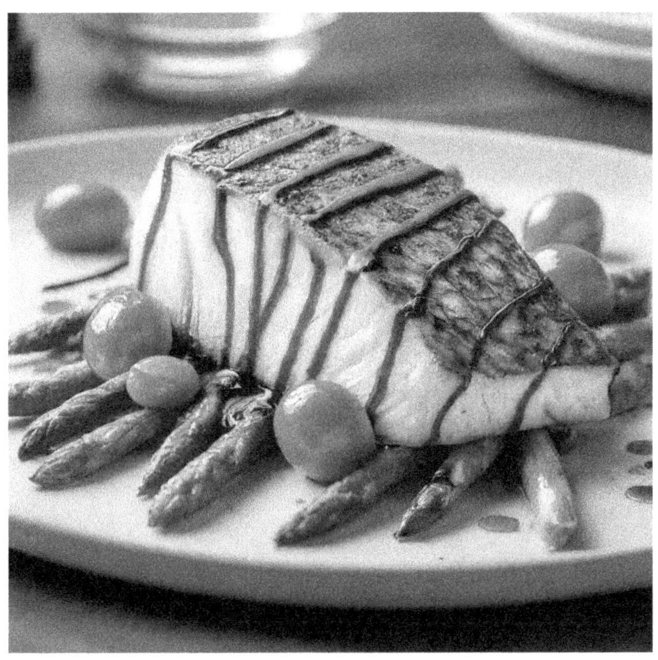

Preparation Time: 5 minutes

Cooking Time: 15-18 minutes

Ingredients:

- 4 (6 Oz) halibut filets

- 2 tbsp. butter, melted

- 1 tsp lemon zest

- 1 tsp salt

- 1/2 tsp black pepper

Instructions:

1. Preheat your oven to 400°F (200°C).

2. Pat the halibut filets dry with paper towels and place them in a baking dish.

3. Brush the halibut filets all over with the melted butter and sprinkle the lemon zest, salt, and black pepper evenly over the top.

4. Bake the halibut for 15-18 minutes, or until it flakes easily with a fork and reaches an internal temperature of 145°F (63°C).

5. Serve the carnivore baked halibut hot.

Nutritional Value (per serving):

- Calories: 240

- Fat: 12g

- Protein: 30g

- Carbohydrates: 0g

50. Carnivore Shrimp Cocktail

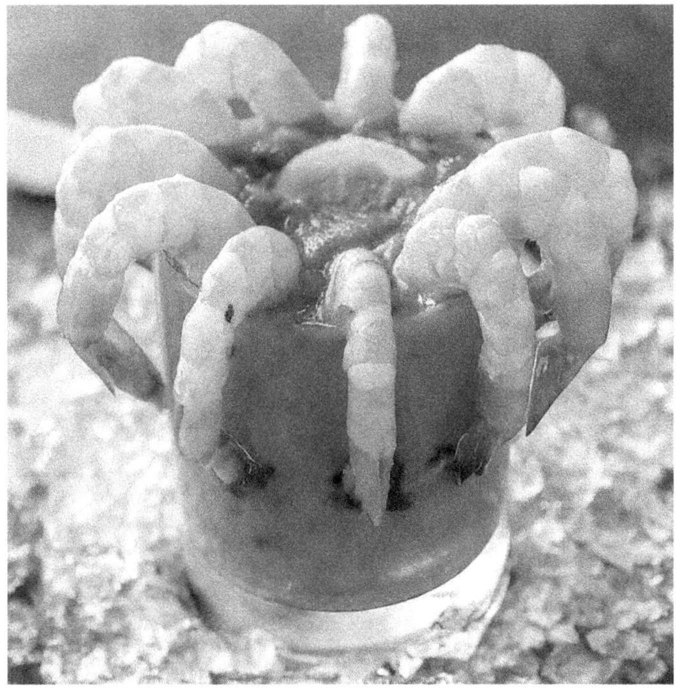

Preparation Time: 10 minutes

Cooking Time: 0 minutes

Ingredients:

- 1 lb. large shrimp, peeled and deveined

- 1/4 cup lemon juice

- 1 tsp salt

- 1/2 tsp black pepper

- Lemon wedges for serving

Instructions:

1. In a large bowl, combine the shrimp, lemon juice, salt, and black pepper. Toss to coat the shrimp evenly.

2. Cover the bowl and refrigerate for at least 30 minutes, or up to 2 hours, to allow the flavors to meld.

3. Arrange the chilled shrimp on a serving platter and serve with lemon wedges.

Nutritional Value (per serving):

- Calories: 120

- Fat: 2g

- Protein: 20g

- Carbohydrates: 2g

CHAPTER 6: Carnivore Diet Salad

51. Carnivore Cobb Salad

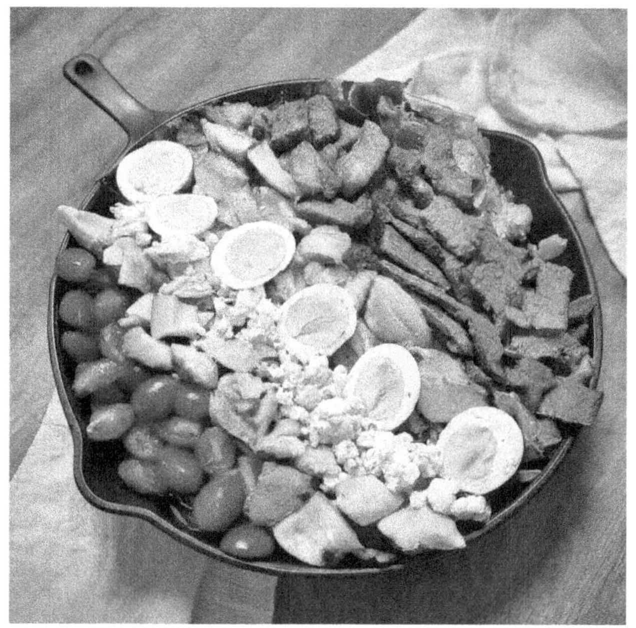

Preparation Time: 20 minutes

Cooking Time: 0 minutes

Ingredients:

- 6 cups mixed greens

- 2 hard-boiled eggs, chopped

- 4 slices bacon, cooked and crumbled

- 1 avocado, diced

- 1 tomato, diced

- 4 Oz grilled chicken breast, diced

- 2 tbsp. blue cheese crumbles

- 2 tbsp. ranch dressing

Instructions:

1. Arrange the mixed greens in a big salad bowl.

2. Top the greens with the chopped hard-boiled eggs, crumbled bacon, diced avocado, diced tomato, diced grilled chicken, and blue cheese crumbles.

3. Pour the dressing evenly over the salad before serving.

Nutritional Value (per serving):
- Calories: 380
- Fat: 28g
- Protein: 28g
- Carbohydrates: 8g

52. Carnivore Steak Salad

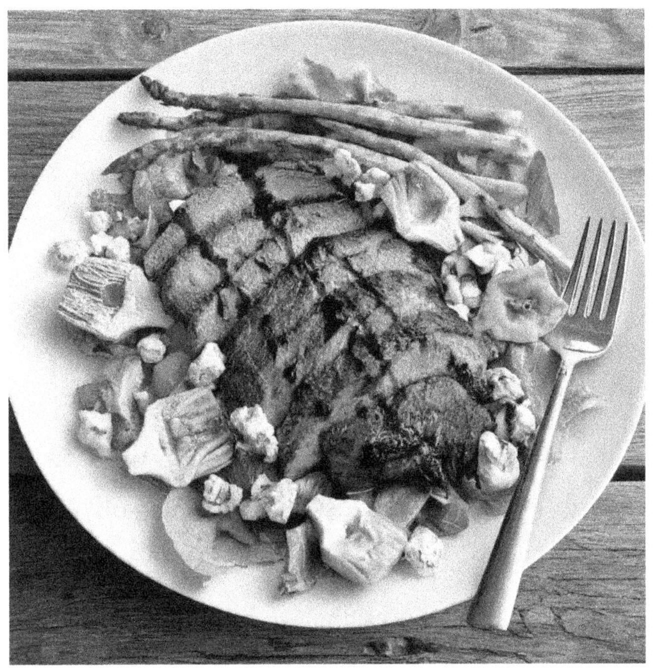

Preparation Time: 15 minutes

Cooking Time: 10 minutes

Ingredients:

- 6 cups mixed greens

- 8 oz grilled or seared steak, sliced

- 1/2 cup cherry tomatoes, halved

- 1/4 cup crumbled blue cheese

- 2 tbsp olive oil

- 1 tbsp balsamic vinegar

- 1 tsp Dijon mustard

- 1/2 tsp salt

- 1/4 tsp black pepper

Instructions:

1. Arrange the mixed greens in a big salad bowl..

2. Top the greens with the sliced grilled or seared steak, cherry tomatoes, and crumbled blue cheese.

3. In a small bowl, whisk together the olive oil, balsamic vinegar, Dijon mustard, salt, and black pepper to make the dressing.

4. Pour the dressing evenly over the salad before serving.

Nutritional Value (per serving):

- Calories: 350

- Fat: 24g

- Protein: 30g

- Carbohydrates: 6g

53. Carnivore Salmon Avocado Salad

Preparation Time: 15 minutes

Cooking Time: 10 minutes

Ingredients:

- 6 cups mixed greens

- 4 Oz grilled or baked salmon, flaked

- 1 avocado, diced

- 1/4 cup sliced cucumber

- 2 tbsp. olive oil

- 1 tbsp. lemon juice

- 1/2 tsp salt

- 1/4 tsp black pepper

Instructions:

1. Arrange the mixed greens in a big salad bowl.

2. Top the greens with the flaked grilled or baked salmon, diced avocado, and sliced cucumber.

3. In a small bowl, whisk together the olive oil, lemon juice, salt, and black pepper to make the dressing.

4. Pour the dressing evenly over the salad before serving.

Nutritional Value (per serving):

- Calories: 320

- Fat: 22g

- Protein: 25g

- Carbohydrates: 8g

54. Carnivore Tuna Nicosia Salad

Preparation Time: 20 minutes

Cooking Time: 10 minutes

Ingredients:

- 6 cups mixed greens

- 4 Oz seared or grilled tuna, sliced

- 2 hard-boiled eggs, quartered

- 1/4 cup black olives, pitted and halved

- 1/2 cup cherry tomatoes, halved

- 2 tbsp. olive oil

- 1 tbsp. red wine vinegar

- 1 tsp Dijon mustard

- 1/2 tsp salt

- 1/4 tsp black pepper

Instructions:

1. Arrange the mixed greens in a big salad bowl.

2. Top the greens with the sliced seared or grilled tuna, quartered hard-boiled eggs, black olive halves, and cherry tomato halves.

3. In a small bowl, whisk together the olive oil, red wine vinegar, Dijon mustard, salt, and black pepper to make the dressing.

4. Pour the dressing evenly over the salad before serving.

Nutritional Value (per serving):

- Calories: 340

- Fat: 22g

- Protein: 30g

- Carbohydrates: 8g

55. Carnivore Chicken Caesar Salad

Preparation Time: 15 minutes
Cooking Time: 10 minutes

Ingredients:

- 6 cups romaine lettuce, chopped

- 4 Oz grilled or roasted chicken, diced

- 2 tbsp. grated Parmesan cheese

- 2 tbsp. Caesar dressing (made with avocado oil and lemon juice)

- 1 tbsp. lemon juice

- 1/2 tsp salt

- 1/4 tsp black pepper

Instructions:

1. In a large salad bowl, combine the chopped romaine lettuce, diced grilled or roasted chicken, and grated Parmesan cheese.

2. In a small bowl, whisk together the Caesar dressing, lemon juice, salt, and black pepper.

3. Drizzle the dressing over the salad and toss to coat the ingredients evenly.

4. Serve the carnivore chicken Caesar salad immediately.

Nutritional Value (per serving):

- Calories: 280

- Fat: 16g

- Protein: 28g

- Carbohydrates: 6g

56. Carnivore Bacon and Egg Salad

Preparation Time: 15 minutes

Cooking Time: 10 minutes

Ingredients:

- 6 cups mixed greens

- 4 hard-boiled eggs, chopped

- 4 slices bacon, cooked and crumbled

- 2 tbsp. avocado oil

- 1 tbsp. apple cider vinegar

- 1 tsp Dijon mustard

- 1/2 tsp salt

- 1/4 tsp black pepper

Instructions:

1. Arrange the mixed greens in a big salad bowl..

2. Top the greens with the chopped hard-boiled eggs and crumbled bacon.

3. In a small bowl, whisk together the avocado oil, apple cider vinegar, Dijon mustard, salt, and black pepper to make the dressing.

4. Pour the dressing evenly over the salad before serving.

Nutritional Value (per serving):

- Calories: 320

- Fat: 24g

- Protein: 20g

- Carbohydrates: 6g

57. Carnivore Shrimp Avocado Salad

Preparation Time: 15 minutes

Cooking Time: 5 minutes

Ingredients:

- 6 cups mixed greens

- 8 Oz cooked shrimp, peeled and deveined

- 1 avocado, diced

- 1/4 cup cherry tomatoes, halved

- 2 tbsp. olive oil

- 1 tbsp. lemon juice

- 1/2 tsp salt

- 1/4 tsp black pepper

Instructions:

1. Arrange the mixed greens in a big salad bowl..

2. Top the greens with the cooked shrimp, diced avocado, and halved cherry tomatoes.

3. In a small bowl, whisk together the olive oil, lemon juice, salt, and black pepper to make the dressing.

4. Pour the dressing evenly over the salad before serving.

Nutritional Value (per serving):

- Calories: 320

- Fat: 22g

- Protein: 25g

- Carbohydrates: 8g

58. carnivore Beef Taco Salad

Preparation Time: 20 minutes

Cooking Time: 10 minutes

Ingredients:

- 6 cups mixed greens

- 8 Oz ground beef, cooked and crumbled

- 1/4 cup shredded cheddar cheese

- 2 tbsp. sour cream

- 2 tbsp. guacamole

- 1 tbsp. olive oil

- 1 tbsp. lime juice

- 1/2 tsp chili powder

- 1/4 tsp salt

Instructions:

1. Arrange the mixed greens in a big salad bowl.

2. Top the greens with the cooked and crumbled ground beef, shredded cheddar cheese, sour cream, and guacamole.

3. in a small bowl, whisk together the olive oil, lime juice, chili powder, and salt to make the dressing.

4. Pour the dressing evenly over the salad before serving.

Nutritional Value (per serving):

- Calories: 360

- Fat: 26g

- Protein: 28g

- Carbohydrates: 8g

59. Carnivore Pork Belly Salad

Preparation Time: 15 minutes
Cooking Time: 20 minutes

Ingredients:

- 6 cups mixed greens

- 8 Oz crispy pork belly, diced

- 1/4 cup cherry tomatoes, halved

- 2 tbsp. blue cheese crumbles

- 2 tbsp. olive oil

- 1 tbsp. apple cider vinegar

- 1 tsp Dijon mustard

- 1/2 tsp salt

- 1/4 tsp black pepper

Instructions:

1. Arrange the mixed greens in a big salad bowl.

2. Top the greens with the diced crispy pork belly, halved cherry tomatoes, and blue cheese crumbles.

3. In a small bowl, whisk together the olive oil, apple cider vinegar, Dijon mustard, salt, and black pepper to make the dressing.

4. Pour the dressing evenly over the salad before serving.

Nutritional Value (per serving):

- Calories: 340

- Fat: 26g

- Protein: 22g

- Carbohydrates: 6g

60. Carnivore Spinach Salad with Bacon and Eggs

Preparation Time: 15 minutes

Cooking Time: 10 minutes

Ingredients:

- 6 cups baby spinach

- 4 hard-boiled eggs, sliced

- 4 slices bacon, cooked and crumbled

- 2 tbsp. olive oil

- 1 tbsp. red wine vinegar

- 1 tsp Dijon mustard

- 1/2 tsp salt

- 1/4 tsp black pepper

Instructions:

1. In a large salad bowl, arrange the baby spinach.

2. Top the spinach with the sliced hard-boiled eggs and crumbled bacon.

3. In a small bowl, whisk together the olive oil, red wine vinegar, Dijon mustard, salt, and black pepper to make the dressing.

4. Pour the dressing evenly over the salad before serving.

Nutritional Value (per serving):

- Calories: 300

- Fat: 22g

- Protein: 18g

- Carbohydrates: 6g

CHAPTER 7: Carnivore Diet Snacks

61. Carnivore Beef Jerky

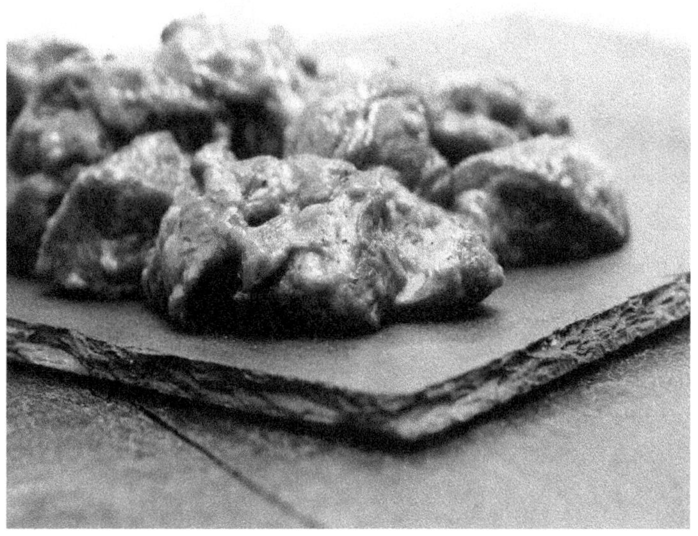

Preparation Time: 20 minutes

Cooking Time: 4-6 hours

Ingredients:

- 2 lbs. beef flank steak or top round, sliced into 1/4-inch thick strips

- 2 tbsp. salt

- 1 tbsp. black pepper

- 1 tsp garlic powder

- 1 tsp onion powder

Instructions:

1. Pat the beef strips dry with paper towels and place them in a large bowl.

2. In a small bowl, mix the salt, black pepper, garlic powder, and onion powder.

3. Sprinkle the spice mixture over the beef strips and toss to coat them evenly.

4. Arrange the seasoned beef strips in a single layer on dehydrator trays or a baking sheet lined with a wire rack.

5. Dehydrate the beef jerky in a dehydrator at 155°F (68°C) for 4-6 hours, or until the jerky is dry and leathery, but still pliable.

6. Alternatively, you can bake the jerky in a preheated 175°F (80°C) oven for 4-6 hours, flipping the strips halfway through.

7. Store the carnivore beef jerky in an airtight container at room temperature for up to 2 weeks.

Nutritional Value (per serving):

- Calories: 120

- Fat: 4g

- Protein: 18g

- Carbohydrates: 0g

62. Carnivore Pork Rinds

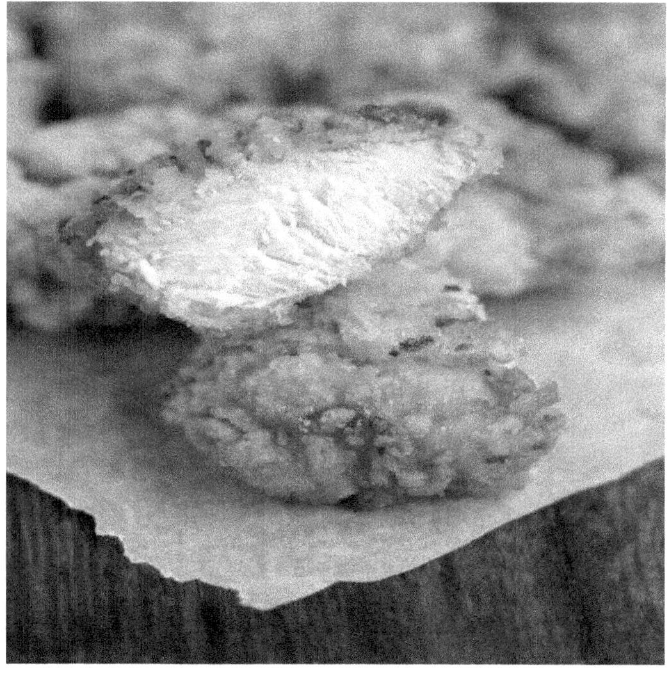

Preparation Time: 10 minutes

Cooking Time: 15-20 minutes

Ingredients:

- 1 lb pork skin, with fat attached

- 1 tsp salt

Instructions:

1. Preheat your oven to 400°F (200°C).

2. Pat the pork skin dry with paper towels and cut it into 1-inch pieces.

3. Arrange the pork skin pieces in a single layer on a baking sheet.

4. Sprinkle the salt evenly over the pork skin.

5. Bake for 15-20 minutes, or until the pork rinds are puffed and golden brown.

6. Allow the carnivore pork rinds to cool completely before serving.

Nutritional Value (per serving):

- Calories: 150

- Fat: 10g

- Protein: 15g

- Carbohydrates: 0g

63. Carnivore Deviled Eggs

Preparation Time: 15 minutes

Cooking Time: 0 minutes

Ingredients:

- 6 hard-boiled eggs, peeled

- 2 tbsp. mayonnaise

- 1 tsp Dijon mustard

- 1/4 tsp salt

- 1/8 tsp black pepper

- Paprika for garnish (optional)

Instructions:

1. Cut the hard-boiled eggs in half lengthwise and carefully remove the yolks, placing them in a small bowl.

2. In the bowl with the yolks, mash them with a fork and mix in the mayonnaise, Dijon mustard, salt, and black pepper until well combined.

3. Spoon or pipe the yolk mixture back into the egg white halves.

4. Sprinkle the deviled eggs with paprika for garnish, if desired.

5. Serve the carnivore deviled eggs chilled.

Nutritional Value (per serving):

- Calories: 100

- Fat: 8g

- Protein: 6g

- Carbohydrates: 0g

64. Carnivore Bacon Wrapped Jalapeño Poppers

Preparation Time: 20 minutes
Cooking Time: 20 minutes

Ingredients:

- 6 jalapeño peppers, halved lengthwise and seeded

- 4 oz. cream cheese, softened

- 1/4 cup shredded cheddar cheese

- 6 slices bacon, cut in half

Instructions:

1. Preheat your oven to 400°F (200°C).

2. In a small bowl, mix the softened cream cheese and shredded cheddar cheese.

3. Spoon the cheese mixture into the hollowed-out jalapeño halves.

4. Wrap each stuffed jalapeño half with a half-slice of bacon, securing it with a toothpick.

5. Arrange the bacon-wrapped jalapeño poppers on a baking sheet.

6. Bake for 20 minutes, or until the bacon is crispy.

7. Serve the carnivore bacon-wrapped jalapeño poppers hot.

Nutritional Value (per serving):

- Calories: 120

- Fat: 10g

- Protein: 6g

- Carbohydrates: 2g

65. Carnivore Cheese Crisps

Preparation Time: 5 minutes

Cooking Time: 10-12 minutes

Ingredients:

- 1 cup shredded cheddar cheese

- 1/4 tsp paprika (optional)

Instructions:

1. Preheat your oven to 400°F (200°C).

2. Line a baking sheet with parchment paper.

3. Scoop the shredded cheddar cheese onto the prepared baking sheet, forming small piles about 2 inches apart.

4. Sprinkle the paprika over the cheese piles, if desired.

5. Bake for 10-12 minutes, or until the cheese is melted and the edges are golden brown.

6. Allow the carnivore cheese crisps to cool completely before serving.

Nutritional Value (per serving):

- Calories: 80

- Fat: 6g

- Protein: 6g

- Carbohydrates: 0g

66. Carnivore Salami and Cheese Roll-Ups

Preparation Time: 10 minutes

Cooking Time: 0 minutes

Ingredients:

- 8 slices salami

- 4 slices cheddar cheese

- 2 tbsp. cream cheese, softened

Instructions:

1. Spread a thin layer of cream cheese on each slice of cheddar cheese.

2. Place a slice of salami on top of each cheese slice and roll it up tightly.

3. Secure the roll-ups with toothpicks, if desired.

4. Serve the carnivore salami and cheese roll-ups chilled.

Nutritional Value (per serving):

- Calories: 150

- Fat: 12g

- Protein: 10g

- Carbohydrates: 0g

67. Carnivore Pork Belly Bites

Preparation Time: 10 minutes

Cooking Time: 30-40 minutes

Ingredients:

- 1 lb. pork belly, cut into 1-inch cubes

- 1 tbsp. salt

- 1 tsp black pepper

- 1 tbsp. baking soda

Instructions:

1. Preheat your oven to 400°F (200°C).

2. Pat the pork belly cubes dry with paper towels and place them in a large bowl.

3. Sprinkle the salt, black pepper, and baking soda over the pork belly cubes and toss to coat them evenly.

4. Arrange the seasoned pork belly cubes in a single layer on a baking sheet lined with parchment paper.

5. Roast the pork belly bites for 30-40 minutes, or until they are crispy and golden brown.

6. Serve the carnivore pork belly bites hot.

Nutritional Value (per serving):

- Calories: 220

- Fat: 18g

- Protein: 15g

- Carbohydrates: 0g

68. Carnivore Chicken Liver Pâté

Preparation Time: 15 minutes
Cooking Time: 30 minutes

Ingredients:

- 1 lb. chicken livers, trimmed

- 1/2 cup butter, softened

- 2 tbsp. heavy cream

- 1 tsp salt

- 1/2 tsp black pepper

- 1/4 tsp ground nutmeg

Instructions:

1. In a large skillet, cook the chicken livers over medium-high heat for 5-7 minutes, or until they are cooked through and no longer pink. Allow to cool slightly.

2. In a food processor, combine the cooked chicken livers, softened butter, heavy cream, salt, black pepper, and ground nutmeg. Blend until smooth and creamy.

3. Transfer the pâté to a serving dish or ramekins and refrigerate for at least 2 hours, or until firm.

4. Serve the carnivore chicken liver pâté chilled, with additional butter or tallow for dipping.

Nutritional Value (per serving):

- Calories: 280

- Fat: 22g

- Protein: 18g

- Carbohydrates: 1g

69. Carnivore Beef Tallow Fries

Preparation Time: 15 minutes

Cooking Time: 20-25 minutes

Ingredients:

- 2 lbs. beef tallow

- 2 lbs. beef fat, cut into 1/2-inch thick fry-shaped pieces
- 1 tsp salt

Instructions:

1. In a large, heavy-bottomed pot or Dutch oven, heat the beef tallow to 375°F (190°C).

2. Working in batches, carefully add the beef fat pieces to the hot tallow and fry for 20-25 minutes, or until golden brown and crispy.

3. Using a slotted spoon, transfer the carnivore beef tallow fries to a paper towel-lined plate.

4. Sprinkle the hot fries with the salt.

5. Serve the carnivore beef tallow fries immediately.

Nutritional Value (per serving):

- Calories: 280
- Fat: 28g
- Protein: 0g
- Carbohydrates: 0g

70. Carnivore Beef Bone Broth Gummies

Preparation Time: 10 minutes

Cooking Time: 15 minutes

Ingredients:

- 2 cups beef bone broth

- 4 tbsp. grass-fed gelatin powder

- 1 tsp vanilla extract (optional)

Instructions:

1. In a small saucepan, whisk together the beef bone broth and gelatin powder until the gelatin is fully dissolved.

2. Heat the mixture over medium heat, stirring constantly, until it just begins to simmer.

3. Remove the pan from the heat and stir in the vanilla extract, if using.

4. Carefully pour the mixture into silicone gummy molds or a baking dish.

5. Refrigerate the carnivore beef bone broth gummies for at least 2 hours, or until firm.

6. Carefully remove the gummies from the molds or cut them into cubes if using a baking dish.

7. Store the carnivore beef bone broth gummies in an airtight container in the refrigerator for up to 1 week.

Nutritional Value (per serving):

- Calories: 50

- Fat: 0g

- Protein: 10g

- Carbohydrates: 0g

CONCLUSION

As you near the conclusion of this beginner's guide to the carnivore diet, you've embarked on a voyage to unlock the transformative essence of meat-centered eating.

Within these pages, you've encountered the straightforwardness, fulfillment, and delectability that characterize the carnivore way of life. From succulent cuts of meat to hearty stews, each recipe has been meticulously crafted to excite your palate and fuel your body from within.

Yet, beyond the culinary escapades and health benefits lies a deeper truth: the carnivore diet embodies more than just a dietary preference—it embodies a philosophy, a mindset, and a return to our primal instincts.

By embracing the carnivore lifestyle, you're not merely feeding your body with nourishing foods; you're reclaiming your well-being, vitality, and connection to nature.

As you progress along your carnivore journey, understand that success isn't about perfection but about growth. Grant yourself grace and adaptability as you navigate this new eating approach. Listen to your body's signals, honor your cravings, and have faith in your innate instincts. With each meal, each mouthful, you're nurturing not only your body but also your spirit, reclaiming your natural place as a carnivore.

Therefore, to you, esteemed reader, I present this special encouragement: dare to embrace the carnivore lifestyle with bravery and certainty. Release apprehension, uncertainty, and societal standards, and have confidence in your body's inherent wisdom. Whether you're pursuing better health, enhanced performance, or simply a deeper connection to your primal essence, the carnivore diet offers a pathway to reviving your vitality and unlocking your full potential.

May this guidebook serve as a compass, a companion, and a wellspring of motivation on your carnivore voyage? May each recipe, each meal, remind you of the abundance, the straightforwardness, and the delight that arises from nourishing your body with its ideal sustenance. Embrace the carnivore lifestyle with an open mind and a ravenous spirit, and observe as it not only revolutionizes you're eating habits but also enriches your life.

MEAL PLAN

Day 1

Breakfast: Carnivore Breakfast Sandwich

Lunch: Carnivore Chicken Salad

Dinner: Carnivore Roasted Chicken

Snack: Carnivore Beef Jerky

Day 2

Breakfast: Carnivore Fat Bomb Fluffy Egg & Cheese Muffins

Lunch: Carnivore Ribeye Steak

Dinner: Carnivore Beef Stroganoff

Snack: Carnivore Pork Rinds

Day 3

Breakfast: Carnivore Quiche

Lunch: Carnivore Chicken Wings

Dinner: Carnivore Beef Chili

Snack: Carnivore Deviled Eggs

Day 4

Breakfast: Carnivore Breakfast Burrito

Lunch: Carnivore Grilled Salmon

Dinner: Carnivore Beef Brisket

Snack: Carnivore Cheese Crisps

Day 5

Breakfast: Carnivore Breakfast Skillet

Lunch: Carnivore Shrimp Scampi

Dinner: Carnivore Lamb Chops

Snack: Carnivore Salami and Cheese Roll-Ups

Day 6

Breakfast: Carnivore Breakfast Meatballs

Lunch: Carnivore Seared Scallops

Dinner: Carnivore Chicken Thighs with Crispy Skin

Snack: Carnivore Chicken Liver Pâté

Day 7

Breakfast: Carnivore Breakfast Sausage Patties

Lunch: Carnivore Pork Belly

Dinner: Carnivore Beef Stew

Snack: Carnivore Beef Tallow Fries

Day 8

Breakfast: Carnivore Breakfast Tacos

Lunch: Carnivore Tuna Nicosia Salad

Dinner: Carnivore Beef Meatballs

Snack: Carnivore Bacon Wrapped Jalapeño Poppers

Day 9

Breakfast: Carnivore Breakfast Salmon Roll-Ups

Lunch: Carnivore Seared Ahi Tuna

Dinner: Carnivore Chicken Parmesan

Snack: Carnivore Pork Belly Bites

Day 10

Breakfast: Carnivore Breakfast Steak and Eggs

Lunch: Carnivore Cobb Salad

Dinner: Carnivore Baked Cod

Snack: Carnivore Beef Bone Broth Gummies

Day 11

Breakfast: Carnivore Chicken Caesar Salad

Lunch: Carnivore Crab Cakes

Dinner: Carnivore Pork Chops

Snack: Carnivore Beef Jerky

Day 12

Breakfast: Carnivore Spinach Salad with Bacon and Eggs

Lunch: Carnivore Baked Halibut

Dinner: Carnivore Lamb Meatballs

Snack: Carnivore Pork Rinds

Day 13

Breakfast: Carnivore Bacon and Egg Salad

Lunch: Carnivore Shrimp Cocktail

Dinner: Carnivore Pork Sausage

Snack: Carnivore Cheese Crisps

Day 14

Breakfast: Carnivore Breakfast Skillet

Lunch: Carnivore Salmon Avocado Salad

Dinner: Carnivore Beef Stroganoff

Snack: Carnivore Deviled Eggs

This meal plan provides a variety of carnivore-friendly meals and snacks, ensuring a balanced and enjoyable diet over 14 days.